Use of Patented Traditional Chinese Medicine against COVID-19

A Practical Manual

Other Related Titles from World Scientific

COVID-19 from Traditional Chinese Medicine Perspective:
Severe Clinical Cases in the Context of Syndrome Differentiation
by Luqi Huang, Hao Li, Wensheng Qi, Zhixu Yang and Qing Miao
ISBN: 978-981-122-874-2

Hydrogen-Oxygen Inhalation for Treatment of COVID-19:
With Commentary from Zhong Nanshan
by Kecheng Xu
ISBN: 978-981-122-329-7

The Key to Healthy Living: A COVID-19 Warrior Talks About Health
by Nanshan Zhong
ISBN: 978-981-123-680-8
ISBN: 978-981-123-748-5 (pbk)

Traditional Chinese and Western Medicine for Diagnosis and Treatment
of Coronavirus Disease 2019 (COVID-19)
edited by Boli Zhang and Qingquan Liu
ISBN: 978-981-122-805-6

Use of Patented Traditional Chinese Medicine against COVID-19

A Practical Manual

Editors

Huaqiang Zhai
Beijing University of Chinese Medicine, China

Yanping Wang
Institute of Basic Research in Clinical Medicine,
China Academy of Chinese Medical Sciences, China

Yiheng Yang
Peking University Third Hospital, China

Xiaodong Li
Hubei Provincial Hospital of Traditional Chinese Medicine, China

Yingjun Shao
Beijing University of Chinese Medicine, China

Chemical Industry Press

World Scientific

NEW JERSEY · LONDON · SINGAPORE · BEIJING · SHANGHAI · HONG KONG · TAIPEI · CHENNAI · TOKYO

Published by

World Scientific Publishing Co. Pte. Ltd.
5 Toh Tuck Link, Singapore 596224
USA office: 27 Warren Street, Suite 401-402, Hackensack, NJ 07601
UK office: 57 Shelton Street, Covent Garden, London WC2H 9HE

and

Chemical Industry Press
No. 13, Qingnianhu South Street
Dongcheng District, Beijing 100011
P. R. China

British Library Cataloguing-in-Publication Data
A catalogue record for this book is available from the British Library.

USE OF PATENTED TRADITIONAL CHINESE MEDICINE AGAINST COVID-19
A Practical Manual

ISBN 978-981-122-787-5 (hardcover)
ISBN 978-981-122-788-2 (ebook for institutions)
ISBN 978-981-122-789-9 (ebook for individuals)

DISCLAIMER: To the extent permissible under applicable laws, no responsibility is assumed by World Scientific nor by Chemical Industry Press for any injury and/or damage to persons or property as a result of any actual or alleged libellous statements, infringement of intellectual property or privacy rights, or products liability, whether resulting from negligence or otherwise, or from any use or operation of any ideas, instructions, procedures, products or methods contained in the material therein.

For any available supplementary material, please visit
https://www.worldscientific.com/worldscibooks/10.1142/12029#t=suppl

Typeset by Stallion Press
Email: enquiries@stallionpress.com

Preface

Coronavirus Disease 2019 (COVID-19) is a severe and complex epidemic that has been ravaging many countries and regions. In January 2020, the WHO announced that the COVID-19 outbreak was a "public health emergency of international concern". Traditional Chinese medicine (TCM) has accumulated rich experience and achieved outstanding effects in its struggle against epidemics for thousands of years. As an essential intervention for prevention and control of COVID-19, TCM boasts significant effects in relieving fever symptoms, slowing down disease progression, preventing disease transformation, reducing steroid dosage, and alleviating complications. Establishing and improving the emergency supply service mode of Chinese medicine in response to public health emergencies and scientifically managing and allocating Chinese medicine resources are conducive to establishing a green channel for the emergency supply of Chinese medicine in response to major public health emergencies in China.

The White Paper entitled "Fighting COVID-19 China in Action", released by the State Council Information Office, PRC, contains certain statistics regarding the use of traditional Chinese medicine: 92% confirmed cases infected with COVID-19 have been treated with traditional Chinese medicine. The performance of traditional Chinese medicine in major public health events has attracted wide attention of the international community. Based on the 7th Trial Version of the Guidelines for the Diagnosis and Treatment of COVID-19 by the National Health Commission and National Administration of Traditional Chinese Medicine of China, this book focuses on the four oral Chinese patent medicines* [Huoxiang Zhengqi capsule (pill, oral liquid, water), Jinhua Qinggan granule, Lianhua Qingwen capsule (granule), and Shufeng Jiedu capsule (granule)] used in the medical observation period and eight TCM injections (Xiyanping injection, Tanreqing injection, Xuebijing injection, Reduning injection, Xingnaojing injection, Shengmai injection, Shenfu injec-tion, and Shenmai injection) used in the clinical treatment period, highlighting the actions, indications, mixed administration, side effects, and pharmacological actions of these twelve Chinese patent medicines while giving full consideration to pharmacists' notes in ensuring the safety and rational use of Chinese patent medicine. This work is not only an important part of the theoretical system of TCM treatment based on syndrome differentiation but also an effective way to promote an even deeper integration of clinical pharmaceutical service and clinical medical practice. Strengthening drug consultation, rational intervention, safety evaluation, post-medication care, setting up a clini-cal pharmaceutical care support team for epidemic prevention and con-trol, and forming a "physician–pharmacologist–patient" whole-course pharmaceutical care emergency response system can effectively facili-tate efficient communication, guarantee the quality of clinical treatment, reduce the occurrence of adverse events in patients, and strengthen the capability of prevention and control of epidemics.

Recent years have witnessed a growing momentum in the develop-ment of the clinical pharmaceutical care of TCM. For the sake of better inheritance and innovation of TCM, it is an essential prerequisite that the original thinking of TCM, the TCM resource treasure house, be integrated with international advanced science and technology. On June 2, President Xi Jinping addressed a group of experts and scholars at a symposium that as a major feature in the prevention and control of COVID-19, the com-bined use of Traditional Chinese medicine and western medicine repre-sents a vivid demonstration of both the inheritance of the tradition and the innovation in the contemporary development of TCM. TCM has gradually grown into more of a new force in the battle than a mere participant in the emergency response, and is now serving as a pioneer in the normal pre-vention and control of COVID-19. This book has been reviewed by Mr. Wang Yongyan, academician of the Chinese Academy of Engineering and honorary President of China Academy of Chinese Medical Sciences, and

---

* "Chinese patent medicine" means the same as "Patented traditional Chinese medicine". For ease of reading, Chinese patent medicine is used in the following paragraphs.

it is recommended by Mr. Jin Shiyuan, master of Chinese medicine and one of the founders of the discipline of Chinese materia medica. The compilation process has been highly valued and supported by the directors of the participating units. The editorial committee is composed of experienced experts engaged in clinical practice, teaching, and research of clinical pharmacy in more than 30 medical colleges and research institutions of China. Relying on the TCM dispensing standardization research center of Beijing University of Chinese medicine, which has made some progress in a series of standard studies on clinical pharmacy, such as the inheritance and innovation of materia medica dispensing, standardization of clinical rational use of materia medica, materia medica quality grading, and the production and processing of materia medica, this editorial committee has utilized data analysis and literature research to sort out the medication law in the use of TCM in COVID-19, and has analyzed and elaborated on the safety of drug use.

In face of the ravaging COVID-19, China has joined hands with other countries to overcome difficulties and contributed wisdom and strength to the global fight against this epidemic. In an open, transparent and responsible manner, China have been proactively fulfilling our international obligations by promptly releasing information on the epidemic and the novel coronavirus gene sequence, reporting the treatment and prevention plans to the World Health Organization (WHO), relevant countries and regional organizations. China has held more than 70 exchange conferences on epidemic prevention and control with many countries and international organizations while sharing its experience in prevention and treatment without reservation through an online knowledge center . Despite having been under great pressure from epidemic prevention and control, China has been providing continuous aid to the international community, including a total of $50 million cash donation to the WHO, 34 medical expert groups dispatched to 32 countries, 283 batches of anti-epidemic aid provided to 150 countries and 4 international organizations, and epidemic prevention materials exported to more than 200 countries and regions. From 15 March to 6 September, a total of 151.5 billion masks, 1.4 billion protective clothing, 230 million goggles, 209,000 respirators, 470 million test kits, and 80.14 million infrared thermometers have been exported to support the global epidemic control and prevention. China calls for the joint efforts in the construction of a human health community and has put forward a series of proposals on international aid and the use of vaccines. With substantial actions, China has helped save tens of thousands of lives around the world, which has demonstrated China's sincere desire to promote the construction of a community with a shared future for mankind!

The compilation of this book has been funded by the National Key R&D Program of China (2019YFC1712000)–Development of international standards for services in clinical pharmaceutical affairs of Chinese Patent Medicine and dispensing education (2019YFC1712002). Special thanks should be hereby conveyed to the scholars who have participated in the compilation, proofreading, and collation of this book! The ancient Chinese proverb goes, "proofreading books is like sweeping fallen leaves, each sweeping tends to be encountered with new leaves." Despite the immense effort made in the compilation of this book, there may inevitably be some omissions. We are looking forward to your comments on possible corrections and valuable suggestions.

Huaqiang Zhai
Chief Editor
April 2020

ABOUT THE EDITORS-IN-CHIEF

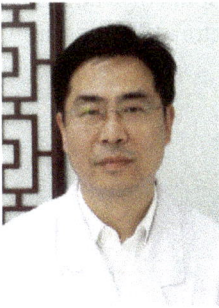

Huaqiang Zhai
Email: jz711@qq.com
Professor and doctoral supervisor of TCM; materia medica experts of ISO(ISO/TC 249); director of several academic associations and winner of several national and provincial awards. Mainly engaged in Chinese medicine standardization, Chinese medicine dispensing technology research.

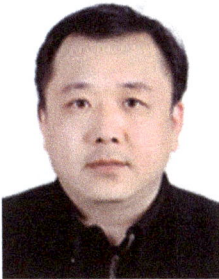

Yanping Wang
Deputy director of Institute of Basic Research in Clinical Medicine, China Academy of Chinese Medical Sciences; deputy secretary-general of two committees of World Federation of Chinese Medicine Societies; director of several academic associations and winner of several national and provincial awards. Mainly engaged in Chinese medicine clinical pharmacy and standardization research and Chinese medicine culture construction and academic heritage research.

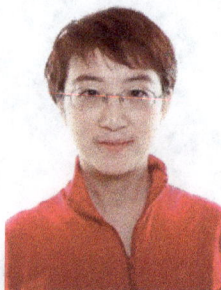

Yiheng Yang
Senior pharmacist and associate supervisor of pharmaceutical preparation section, Peking University Third Hospital. Mainly engaged in pharmaceutical management, pharmaceutical quality control, Chinese medicine clinical pharmacy and post-marketing drug safety evaluation.

Xiaodong Li
Professor, postdoctor, doctoral supervisor; vice-president of Hubei Provincial Hospital of Traditional Chinese Medicine (TCM); director of Hepatology Institute of TCM.

Yingjun Shao
Email:15210369502@163.com.
Postgraduate supervisor, associate professor of translation & interpretation, Beijing University of Chinese Medicine.

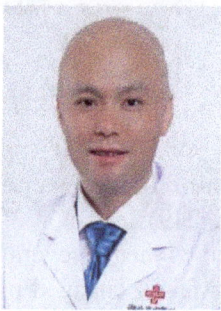

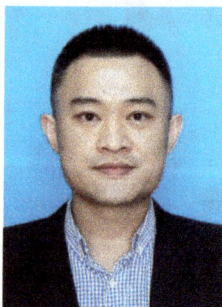

Editorial Board

Guoxiu Liu (Beijing University of Chinese Medicine)

Hongli Wang (Gansu Provincial Hospital of Traditional Chinese Medicine)

Hongshun Wang (Affiliated Hospital of Jiangxi University of Traditional Chinese Medicine)

Hua Nian (Yueyang Hospital of Integrated Traditional Chinese and Western Medicine, Shanghai University of Traditional Chinese Medicine)

Hua Wang (Changchun Hospital of Traditional Chinese Medicine)

Huaqiang Zhai (Beijing University of Chinese Medicine)

Huarong Li (Jingzhou Central Hospital)

Huarong Li (Union Hospital, Tongji Medical College, Huazhong University of Science and Technology)

Huiqing Zhang (Naval Medical University)

Jiankun Wu (Beijing Hospital of Traditional Chinese Medicine, Capital Medical University)

Jiao Liu (Beijing University of Chinese Medicine)

Jie Tian (Ningxia Chinese Medicine Research Center)

Jing Yu (Xinjiang Medical University)

Jingzhou Zhang (Affiliated Hospital of Changchun University of Traditional Chinese Medicine)

Jinsong Yan (Hubei Provincial Hospital of Traditional Chinese Medicine)

Jun Qin (The Second Affiliated Hospital of Guangzhou University of Chinese Medicine)

Junjun Chen (Shanghai Jiao Tong University Affiliated Sixth People's Hospital)

JunLi An (Beijing Children's Hospital Affiliated to Capital Medical University)

Li Liu (Hospital of Chengdu University of Traditional Chinese Medicine)

Li Liu (Shuguang Hospital Affiliated to Shanghai University of Traditional Chinese Medicine)

Li Wang (Beijing Hospital of Traditional Chinese Medicine, Capital Medical University)

Lihua Li (The First Affiliated Hospital of Anhui University of Traditional Chinese Medicine)

Ling Ma (Zhongnan Hospital of Wuhan University)

Lingzhi Zhang (Beijing Anzhen Hospital)

Manqin Yang (The Second Affiliated Hospital of Anhui University of Traditional Chinese Medicine)

Xuanzhong Tan (Nanjing Hospital of Chinese Medicine Affiliated to Nanjing University of Chinese Medicine)

Xuemei Chen (Xiamen Hospital of Traditional Chinese Medicine)

Xuesen Wang (Beijing University of Chinese Medicine)

Yanmei Cao (Beijing University of Chinese Medicine)

Yanping Wang (China Academy of Chinese Medical Sciences)

Yanqing Wang (Beijing Children's Hospital, Capital Medical University)

Yi Guan (Beijing Jishuitan Hospital)

Yi Liu (Traditional Chinese Medicine Hospital of Urumqi)

Yiheng Yang (Peking University Third Hospital)

Ying Liu (Peking University Third Hospital)

Ying Zhang (Eye Hospital, China Academy of Traditional Chinese Medicine)

Yingjun Shao (Beijing University of Chinese Medicine)

Yiran Cui (Beijing Hospital of Traditional Chinese Medicine, Capital Medical University)

Yongjun Li (Zhongda Hospital, Southeast University)

Yonglong Han (Shanghai Jiao Tong University Affiliated Sixth People's Hospital)

Yuanshen Zhu (The First Hospital of Tsinghua University)

Yufei Feng (People's Hospital of Peking University)

Zhengde Huang (Hubei Provincial Hospital of Traditional Chinese Medicine)

Zinan Qin (Beijing University of Chinese Medicine)

Contents

Chapter 1

Understanding COVID-19

Since December 2019, multiple cases of a novel coronavirus pneumonia had been reported in Wuhan City, Hubei Province of China. As the pandemic spread to other areas, such cases were also found in other regions in China as well as countries all over the world. It has been confirmed to be an acute respiratory epidemic disease caused by the infection of a novel coronavirus.

Section 1: Understanding of COVID-19 in Modern Medicine

I. Basic Facts

1. *Terminology*

The new coronavirus pneumonia is referred to as novel coronary pneumonia, whose pathogen is a new coronavirus. The World Health Organization (WHO) has named the new coronavirus pneumonia COVID-19 (Corona Virus Disease 2019). The disease was categorized as an acute respiratory infectious disease on January 20, 2020, and was included in the Class B infectious disease as stipulated in the Law of the People's Republic of China on the Prevention and Control of Infectious Diseases, and was managed as a Class A infectious disease.

2. *Pathogenic characteristics*

The novel coronaviruses belong to the β genus. Their genetic characteristics are significantly different from SARS-CoV and MERS-CoV. Current research has shown that they share more than 85% homology with bat SARS-like coronaviruses (bat-SL-CoVZC45). The new coronavirus is a positive-strand RNA virus.

The virus is sensitive to ultraviolet and heat, which can be effectively inactivated when exposed to 56°C for 30 minutes and lipid solvents (such as ether, 75% ethanol, chlorine-containing disinfectant, peracetic acid, and chloroform). Chlorhexidine has not been effective in inactivating the virus.

II. Epidemiological Characteristics

1. *Source of infection*

The primary source of infection is patients infected with the new coronavirus. Asymptomatic infection may also become a source of infection, and the infectivity of patients at incubation and convalescence stages needs to be further clarified.

Recessive infections may also become a source of infection, which have not been observed in severe acute respiratory syndrome (SARS). Recessively infected people have no symptoms, are difficult to diagnose and quarantine in time, and are more likely to cause the accumulation of infected people in the community, which makes it more difficult to control disease transmission.

2. *Transmission route*

Transmission through respiratory tract droplets and close contact is the main transmission route. In a relatively closed environment, there is a possibility of spreading through aerosols when exposed to high-concentration aerosols for a long time.

(1) Respiratory droplet transmission:
This is the main route of spreading the new coronavirus. The virus spreads through droplets generated when a patient coughs, sneezes, or talks, and the susceptible person inhales the droplets and becomes infected.

(2) Intimate contact transmission:
This means that droplets containing the virus are deposited on the article's surface, which can contaminate the exposed hand, resulting in further infection of the mucous membrane of the mouth, nasal cavity, and eyes.

(3) Aerosol transmission:
Aerosol refers to the nucleus composed of proteins and pathogens, which is formed after the droplets lose water during air suspension. The aerosol can float to a distant place, causing long-distance transmission. There is a possibility of aerosol transmission when exposed to viral aerosols in a closed environment for a long time. There is no evidence that the coronavirus can be transmitted remotely through aerosols.

(4) Digestive tract dissemination:
Although the coronavirus has been detected in the stools of diagnosed patients, indicating that the virus can be replicated and present in the digestive tract, it is not definite whether there is a fecal-oral transmission route.

3. *Susceptible population*

Humans of all ages are generally susceptible. The elderly and those with underlying diseases may develop severe conditions after infection, and the symptoms of children are relatively mild.

Patients with COVID-19 and close contacts of asymptomatic infected cases are populations at high risk of infection. As medical staff and patients' family members treat, care, accompany, and visit the patients, they have more close contact with patients, so their risk of infection is higher.

III. Clinical Features

1. *Clinical manifestations*

The main manifestations of the disease are fever, dry cough, and fatigue. Some patients have mild onset symptoms, even no apparent fever, and may be accompanied by anorexia, nausea, vomiting, and muscle pain in the limbs or the small of the back. With the progress of the disease, dyspnea and (or) hypoxemia gradually appears in a week after the onset. Severe patients may have acute respiratory distress syndrome, septic shock, metabolic acidosis, and coagulation dysfunction. Patients with mild symptoms only show low-grade fever and slight asthenia without signs of pneumonia.

It is worth noting that severe and critical patients in the course of the disease can show low fever or even no obvious fever. Based on the current epidemiological survey, the incubation period is 1–14 days, mostly 3–7 days.

Based on current cases treated, most patients have a good prognosis, and a few patients are in critical condition.

2. *Auxiliary tests*

(1) Laboratory examination:
At the early stage of the disease, the total number of peripheral blood leucocyte (PBL) of patients is normal or decreased, while the lymphocyte count (LC) is reduced. Some patients may have elevated liver enzymes, lactate dehydrogenase (LDH), creatase, and myoglobin. Some severe patients may have increased troponin. Most patients' C-reactive protein (CRP) and erythrocyte sedimentation rate (ESR) increase, while the procalcitonin appears normal. In severe cases, D-dimer increases, and peripheral blood lymphocytes reduce progressively. Severe and critical patients often have elevated inflammatory factors.

Corona Virus nucleic acids can be detected in specimens such as nasopharyngeal swabs, sputum, lower respiratory tract secretions, blood, and feces.

(2) Chest imaging:
In the early stage, imaging shows multiple small, patchy shadows and interstitial changes, which are apparent in the peripheral zone of the lungs. As the disease progresses, imaging shows multiple ground-glass opacities and infiltration in both lungs. In severe cases, pulmonary consolidation may occur, while the pleural effusion is rare.

3. *Diagnostic criteria*

3.1. *Suspected cases*

A comprehensive analysis combined with the following epidemiological history and clinical manifestations should be made to diagnose the suspected cases.

(1) Epidemiological history:
    (a) History of traveling or residence in Wuhan city, surrounding areas, or other communities with reported cases within 14 days before onset.
    (b) Contact history of infected patients (a positive nucleic acid test result) within 14 days before onset.
    (c) Contact history with patients with fever or respiratory symptoms from Wuhan city, surrounding areas, or communities with reported cases within 14 days before onset.
    (d) Clustering occurrence of cases.
(2) Clinical manifestations:
    (a) Fever and (or) respiratory symptoms.
    (b) The imaging features of COVID-19 mentioned above.
    (c) The total number of white blood cells and the lymphocyte count are normal or decreased in the early stage of the disease.

Suspected case: Patients who satisfy any one of the epidemiological exposure history criteria as well as any two items in the clinical manifestations. If there is no definite epidemiological history, then three items in the clinical manifestations must be met.

3.2. *Confirmed cases*

The suspected cases with one of the following etiological points of evidence can be diagnosed as confirmed cases.

(1) Real-time fluorescence RT-PCR detection shows positive results of the novel coronavirus nucleic acid.
(2) The results of virus gene sequencing show high homology to the known 2019 coronaviruses.
(3) The coronavirus-specific IgM and IgG antibodies are positive in serum. The coronavirus-specific IgG antibodies in serum change from negative to positive or increase more than four times in the recovery period than the acute stage.

3.3. *Standardized ICD code*

For timely and accurate communication of information about COVID-19, the National Health Commission has formulated "the Corona Virus Disease 2019 Infection ICD Code"; see Table 1 for details.

Table 1.   The new coronavirus infection-related ICD code.

No.	ICD-10 code	Code Name	Code Description
1.	U07.100	2019 Coronavirus disease	Statistical code
2.	U07.100 × 001	Coronavirus disease	A main diagnosis code; Applicable to inpatients diagnosed with new coronavirus pneumonia
3.	U07.100 × 002	New coronavirus infection	A main diagnosis code; Applicable to inpatients diagnosed with infection (excluding new coronavirus pneumonia)
4.	U07.100 × 003	Clinical diagnosis of new coronavirus pneumonia	Applicable to inpatients with the clinical diagnosis of new coronavirus pneumonia in Hubei Province
5.	Z03.800 × 001	Suspected cases of new coronavirus pneumonia	Applicable to inpatients with suspected cases of new coronavirus pneumonia

4. *Clinical classification*

4.1. *Mild cases*

Patients have mild symptoms with no sign of pneumonia on imaging.

4.2. *Common cases*

Patients have fever and respiratory symptoms with radiological findings of pneumonia.

4.3. *Severe cases*

Cases meeting any of the following criteria:

(1) Respiratory distress ($\geq$ 30 breaths/min);
(2) Oxygen saturation $\leq$ 93% at rest;
(3) Arterial partial pressure of oxygen (PaO2)/fraction of inspired oxygen (FiO2) $\leq$ 300 mmHg (1 mmHg = 0.133 kPa).

In high-altitude areas (at an altitude of over 1,000 meters above the sea level), PaO2/FiO2 should be adjusted using the following equation: PaO2/FiO2 × [Atmospheric pressure (mmHg)/760].

Cases with chest imaging that shows obvious lesion progression within 24–48 hours > 50% should be managed as severe cases.

4.4. *Critical cases*

Cases meeting one of the following criteria:

(1) Respiratory failure with mechanical ventilation;
(2) Shock;
(3) Other organ failures requiring ICU monitoring and treatment.

5. *Differential diagnosis*

(1) The mild manifestations of the new coronavirus infection must be distinguished from upper respiratory tract infections caused by other viruses.

(2) COVID-19 needs to be distinguished from other known viral and mycoplasmal pneumonia affected by the influenza virus, adenovirus, and respiratory syncytial virus. Especially for suspected cases, rapid antigen detection and multiple PCR nucleic acid detection should be adopted as far as possible to detect common respiratory pathogens.

(3) COVID-19 should also be distinguished from non-infectious diseases such as vasculitis, dermatomyositis, and organized pneumonia.

Section 2: Understanding COVID-19 in Traditional Chinese Medicine

Fighting against epidemic diseases using traditional Chinese medicine (TCM) has always been an essential theme in the long history of China, and it is indispensable for ensuring the prosperity of the Chinese nation. The Institute of Basic Research In Clinical Medicine, China Academy of Chinese Medical Sciences, as a supporting organization of experts and scientific research groups in fighting against COVID-19 using TCM, has concluded that COVID-19 belongs to the category of plague or pestilence, based on the clinical manifestations of this disease, Wuhan's climatic characteristics, and relevant ancient literature on epidemic diseases.

I. Historical Review

According to the statistics of *China's Epidemic History*, at least 321 large-scale plagues have occurred in China from the Western Han Dynasty to the late Qing Dynasty. During the Yuan, Ming, and Qing Dynasties, the occurrence of epidemics reached a peak in Chinese history. The duration of years with epidemic disease during the Yuan Dynasty (1271–1368) added up to 30 years; this figure jumped to 118 years during the Ming Dynasty (1368–1644) and 134 years during the Qing Dynasty (1644–1911).

More than 3,000 years ago in the Shang Dynasty (1600 B.C.–1046 B.C.), there were written records of the epidemic situation. *Bamboo Slips on Qin Dynasty evacuated from Yunmeng* (*Yunmeng Qin Jian*) recorded that the Qin Dynasty had set up a "refuge" to compel leprosy patients. *The History of Han Dynasty* (*Han Shu*) stated how epidemic diseases were managed in the 2nd Year since the start of the Han Dynasty: *Vacate the premises, establish separate places, and treat them with medicines for the infected people.*

The above records show that the ancient Chinese governments established temporary public hospitals to control epidemics, indicating that China had adopted isolation measures for infectious diseases as early as 2 A.D.

As for the folk anti-epidemic habits of burning incense to avoid filth, sweeping away filth, and disinfecting drinking water, it has a much longer history and is extremely common in folk use. From Zhang Zhongjing's *Treatise on Cold Damage and Miscellaneous Diseases*

(*Shang Han Za Bing Lun*) in the Eastern Han Dynasty to Wu Youke's first monograph of *On Pestilence* (*Wen Yi Lun*) in the Ming Dynasty, TCM has formed a system of preventing and controlling epidemic diseases with relatively comprehensive theory and technical methods.

Since the establishment of a new China in 1949, China's healthcare conditions have greatly improved. However, looking back on public health events after the founding of the People's Republic of China, traditional Chinese medicine has still played its essential role and made remarkable achievements.

II. Disease Name

According to the senior expert panel of the State Administration of Traditional Chinese Medicine, the new Corona Virus Disease 2019 was categorized as pestilence, upon observation of the clinical manifestations of patients in Wuhan, combined with the climate characteristics of Wuhan.

Based on the relevant literature of epidemics in the past, it is considered that cold pestilence is the general term for acute epidemic infectious exogenous diseases caused by an abnormal cold pathogen or epidemic cold toxin, manifested as cold-damp pestilence and cold dryness pestilence. The cold pestilence is characterized by a short spell of exterior cold pattern at onset, followed by the pattern of exterior cold with interior heat. Alternatively, at initial stage, the pattern presented is already exterior cold with interior heat, which can be complicated by other diseases with the progress of disease.

III. Etiology and Pathogenesis

Taking Wuhan's climatic features into consideration, the cause of the disease is dryness-heat followed by cold, or cold-damp pathogens. Abnormal climate permeates the local environment with complicated dryness, heat, dampness, and cold pathogens. Since mid-December 2019, overcast rain and cold and humid air in Wuhan have provided breeding bed for the outbreak.

The clinical manifestations of the patients feature coughing with shortness of breath. It can be seen that the disease is located mainly in the lungs, also in the spleen and stomach, and exterior defensive qi. The basic pathogenesis of this disease is the excessive dampness and coldness accumulating in the lungs, damaging healthy qi, resulting in qi movement obstruction, abnormal ascending and descending qi movement, and depleted source qi.

Specifically, it is mainly caused by epidemic toxins mixed with cold or damp cold entering the body from the mouth and nose. These toxic damp cold dry pathogens invade the airway, bind with latent dryness, and accumulate in the chest, and toxins, dampness, cold, and dry qi hurt the lungs and the qi in the chest, resulting in damaged lung qi and pectoral qi in the chest. The lungs fail to disperse and descend qi; qi movement is disordered and distribution of water and fluids is also out of order.

When pectoral qi cannot help the heart to move blood, the lungs are also filled with stagnant qi. At the terminal lung vessels, qi and blood are both static, failing to move smoothly, and thus producing blood stasis. Static blood, water dampness, and toxin further exacerbate the qi movement disorder, forming a vicious circle.

Disease progression characteristics: In the early stage, the pattern of exterior cold with interior heat and complex of intermingled deficiency and excess is commonly seen. The disease can progress to an exterior and interior excess heat pattern if the patient has yang excess constitution. If the patient has yang deficiency body constitution, the pattern of yang deficiency with congealing cold may occur; if the heat and pathogenic qi reversely transmit to the pericardium, or toxic pathogen sinks internally, the lungs collapse and the critical cases of internal blockage and external collapse could be present.

IV. Treatment by Stages

See *New Coronavirus Pneumonia Diagnosis and Treatment Program (Trial Version 7)* jointly promulgated by the General Office of the National Health Commission and the Office of the State Administration of Traditional Chinese Medicine.

Chapter 2

Diagnosis and Treatment Protocol for Novel Coronavirus Pneumonia

On March 3, 2020, the General offices of the National Health Commission and State Administration of Traditional Chinese Medicine jointly issued the notice of publishing *New Coronavirus Pneumonia Diagnosis and Treatment Program* (Trial Version 7). In the notice, all relevant medical institutions are required to use TCM proactively and strengthen the combination of TCM and Western Medicine (WM). The TCM–WM joint consultation mechanism should be in place to ensure favorable clinical outcomes in the treatment of COVID-19 patients.

Since December 2019, multiple cases of novel coronavirus pneumonia (NCP) have been identified in Wuhan, Hubei. With the spread of the epidemic, such cases have also been found subsequently in other parts of China and other countries. As an acute respiratory infectious disease, NCP has been included in Class B infectious diseases as is stipulated in the Law of the People's Republic of China on Prevention and Treatment of Infectious Diseases and managed as an infectious disease of Class A.

By taking a series of preventive control and medical treatment measures, the rise of the epidemic situation in China has been contained to a certain extent. The epidemic situation has eased in most provinces, but the morbidity and death toll abroad have been on the rise.

With improved understanding of the clinical manifestations and pathology of the disease, and the accumulation of experience in diagnosis and treatment, in order to facilitate the early diagnosis and early treatment of the disease, improve the curative rate, reduce the mortality rate, prevent nosocomial infection as much as possible, and take better precautions against the further transmission caused by imported cases from overseas, *Diagnosis and Treatment Protocol for Novel Coronavirus Pneumonia* (Trial Version 6) has been revised into *Diagnosis and Treatment Protocol for Novel Coronavirus Pneumonia* (Trial Version 7).

I. Etiological Characteristics

The novel coronaviruses belong to the β genus. They have envelopes, and the particles are round or oval, often polymorphic, with the diameter being 60–140 nm. Their genetic characteristics are significantly different from SARS-CoV and MERS-CoV. Current research shows that they share more than 85% homology with bat SARS-like coronaviruses (bat-SL-CoVZC45). When isolated and cultured in vitro, the 2019-nCoV can be found in human respiratory epithelial cells in about 96 hours; however, it takes about 6 days for the virus to be found if isolated and cultured in Vero E6 and Huh-7 cell lines.

Most of the knowledge about the physical and chemical properties of coronavirus comes from the research on SARS-CoV and MERS-CoV. The virus is sensitive to ultraviolet and heat. Exposure to 56°C for 30 minutes and lipid solvents such as ether, 75% ethanol, chlorine-containing disinfectant, peracetic acid, and chloroform can effectively inactivate the virus. Chlorhexidine has not been effective in inactivating the virus.

II. Epidemiological Characteristics

1. *Source of infection*

Currently, the patients infected by the novel coronavirus are the main source of infection; asymptomatic infected people can also be an infectious source.

2. *Route of transmission*

Transmission of the virus happens mainly through respiratory droplets and close contact. There is the possibility of aerosol transmission in a relatively closed environment following a long-time exposure to high concentrations of aerosol. As the novel coronavirus can be isolated in feces and urine, attention should be paid to feces- or urine-contaminated environments that may lead to aerosol or contact transmission.

3. *Susceptible population*

People are generally susceptible.

III. Pathological Changes

Pathological findings from available autopsies and biopsy studies are summarized below.

1. *Lungs*

Variable consolidation is present in the lungs. The alveoli are filled with fluid and fibrin with hyaline membrane formation. Macrophages and many multinucleated syncytial cells are identified within the alveolar exudates. Type II pneumocytes show marked hyperplasia and focal desquamation. Viral inclusions are observed in type II pneumocytes and macrophages. In addition, there is prominent edema and congestion in the alveolar septa, which are infiltrated by monocytes and lymphocytes. Fibrin microthrombi are present. In more severely affected areas, hemorrhage, necrosis, and overt hemorrhagic infarction are seen. Organization of alveolar exudates and interstitial fibrosis are also present.

Detached epithelial cells and mucus are present in the bronchi; sometimes mucus plugs are seen. Hyperventilated alveoli, interrupted alveolar interstitium, and cystic formation are occasionally seen.

By means of electronic microscopy, cytoplasmic 2019-nCoV virions are observed in the bronchial epithelium and type II pneumocytes. Immunostaining reveals 2019-nCoV viral immunoreactivity in some alveolar epithelial cells and macrophages, and RT-PCR confirms the presence of 2019-nCoV nucleic acid.

2. *Spleen, hilar lymph nodes, and bone marrow*

The spleen is markedly atrophic with a decreased number of lymphocytes. Focal hemorrhage and necrosis are present. Macrophage proliferation and phagocytosis are present in the spleen. The sparsity of lymphocytes and focal necrosis is noted in lymph nodes. CD4+ immunohistochemistry and CD8+ immunohistochemistry highlight a decreased number of *T* cells in the spleen and lymph nodes. Myelopoiesis is decreased in the bone marrow.

3. *Heart and blood vessels*

Degenerated or necrosed myocardial cells are present, along with mild infiltration of monocytes, lymphocytes, and/or neutrophils in the cardiac interstitium. Shedding of endothelial cells, endovasculitis, and thrombi is seen in some blood vessels.

4. *Liver and gallbladder*

The liver is dark red and enlarged. Degeneration and focal necrosis of hepatocytes is found, accompanied by the infiltration of neutrophils. The sinusoids are congested. Lymphocytes and histiocytes infiltrate the portal areas. Microthrombi are seen. The gallbladder is prominently distended.

5. *Kidneys*

The kidneys are marked by proteinaceous exudates in the Bowman's capsule around glomeruli, degeneration and shedding of renal tubules' epithelial cells, and hyaline casts. Microthrombi and fibrotic foci are found in the kidney interstitium.

6. *Other organs*

Cerebral hyperemia and edema are present, with degeneration of some neurons. Necrotic foci are noted in the adrenal glands. Degeneration, necrosis, and desquamation of epithelium mucosae of variable degrees are present in the esophagus, stomach, and bowel.

IV. Clinical Characteristics

1. *Clinical manifestations*

Based on the current epidemiological investigation, the incubation period is 1–14 days, mostly 3–7 days.

The main manifestations include fever, fatigue, and dry cough. Nasal congestion, runny nose, sore throat, myalgia, and diarrhea are found in a few cases. Severe patients develop dyspnea and/or hypoxemia one week after onset and may progress rapidly to acute respiratory distress syndrome, septic shock, refractory metabolic acidosis, coagulopathy, multiple organ failure, etc. It is noteworthy that severe and critically ill patients may only present with moderate to low fever or even no fever at all.

Some children and neonatal patients may have atypical symptoms, presented with gastrointestinal symptoms such as vomiting and diarrhea, or only manifested as lethargy and shortness of breath.

The patients with mild symptoms usually do not develop pneumonia, but have low fever and mild fatigue.

Based on our experience, most patients have a good prognosis, and a small percentage of patients end up critically ill. The prognosis for the elderly and patients with chronic underlying diseases is unfavorable. The clinical course of pregnant women with NCP is similar to that of non-pregnant patients of the same age. Symptoms in children are relatively mild.

2. *Laboratory tests*

2.1. *General findings*

In the early stages of the disease, the peripheral WBC count is normal or decreased, and the lymphocyte count is decreased. Some patients have elevated liver enzymes, lactate dehydrogenase (LDH), muscle enzymes, and myoglobin. Elevated troponin is seen in some critically ill patients. Most patients have elevated C-reactive protein and erythrocyte sedimentation rate and normal procalcitonin. In severe cases, D-dimer increases, and peripheral blood lymphocytes progressively decrease. Severe and critically ill patients often have elevated inflammatory factors.

2.2. *Pathogenic and serological findings*

(1) Pathogenic findings: Novel coronavirus nucleic acid can be detected in nasopharyngeal swabs, sputum, lower respiratory tract secretions, blood, feces, and other specimens by using RT-PCR and/or NGS methods. It is more accurate if specimens are obtained from the lower respiratory tract (sputum or air tract extraction). The specimens should be submitted for testing as soon as possible after collection.
(2) Serological findings: NCP virus-specific IgM becomes detectable around 3–5 days after onset; IgG reaches a titration of at least a 4-fold increase during convalescence compared with the acute phase.

3. *Chest imaging*

In the early stage, imaging shows multiple small patchy shadows and interstitial changes, more apparent in the peripheral zone of the lungs. As the disease progresses, imaging shows multiple ground-glass opacities and infiltration in both lungs. In severe cases, pulmonary consolidation may occur. However, pleural effusion is rare.

V. Case Definitions

1. *Suspected cases*

Diagnosis of suspected cases should be made considering both the epidemiological history and clinical manifestations:

1.1. *Epidemiological history*

(1) History of travel to or residence in Wuhan and its surrounding areas, or in other communities where cases have been reported within 14 days prior to the onset of the disease;

(2) In contact with people infected with the novel coronavirus (with positive results for the nucleic acid test) within 14 days prior to the onset of the disease;

(3) In contact with patients who have a fever or respiratory symptoms from Wuhan and its surrounding areas, or from communities where confirmed cases have been reported within 14 days before the onset of the disease;

(4) Clustered cases (2 or more cases with fever and/or respiratory symptoms in a small area such as families, offices, schools, etc., within two weeks).

1.2. *Clinical manifestations*

(1) Fever and (or) respiratory symptoms;

(2) The imaging shows the abovementioned characteristics of NCP;

(3) Normal or decreased WBC count, normal or decreased lymphocyte count in the early stage of onset.

A suspected case should be defined as having any of the epidemiological history plus any two clinical manifestations or all three clinical manifestations if there is no clear epidemiological history.

2. *Confirmed cases*

Suspected cases with one of the following etiological or serological evidence:

(1) Real-time fluorescent RT-PCR indicates positive for new coronavirus nucleic acid;

(2) Viral gene sequence is highly homologous to new coronaviruses;

(3) NCP virus-specific IgM and IgG are detectable in serum; NCP virus-specific IgG is detectable or reaches a titration of at least a 4-fold increase during convalescence compared with the acute phase.

VI. Clinical Classification

1. *Mild cases*

The clinical symptoms are mild, and there is no sign of pneumonia on imaging.

2. *Moderate cases*

Showing fever and respiratory symptoms with radiological findings of pneumonia.

3. *Severe adult cases meeting any of the following criteria*

(1) Respiratory distress ($\geq$ 30 breaths/min);
(2) Finger oxygen saturation $\leq$ 93% at rest;
(3) Arterial partial pressure of oxygen (PaO_2)/fraction of inspired oxygen (FiO_2) $\leqq$ 300 mmHg (1 mmHg = 0.133 kPa).

In high-altitude areas (at an altitude of over 1,000 meters above the sea level), PaO_2/FiO_2 shall be corrected by the following formula: $PaO_2/FiO_2 \times$ [Atmospheric pressure (mmHg)/760].

Cases with chest imaging that shows obvious lesion progression within 24–48 hours: > 50% shall be managed as severe cases.

Child cases meeting any of the following criteria:

(1) Tachypnea (RR $\geq$ 60 breaths/min for infants aged below two months; RR $\geq$ 50 BPM for infants aged 2–12 months; RR $\geq$ 40 BPM for children aged 1–5 years, and RR $\geq$ 30 BPM for children above five years of age) independent of fever and crying;
(2) Oxygen saturation $\leq$ 92% on finger pulse oximeter taken at rest;
(3) Labored breathing (moaning, nasal fluttering, and infrasternal, supraclavicular and intercostal retraction), cyanosis, and intermittent apnea;
(4) Somnolence and convulsion;
(5) Difficulty in feeding and signs of dehydration.

4. *Critical cases*

Cases meeting any of the following criteria:

(1) Respiratory failure requiring mechanical ventilation;
(2) Shock;
(3) With other organ failures that require ICU care.

VII. Early Clinical Warning Indicators of Severe and Critical Cases

1. *Adults*

(1) The peripheral blood lymphocytes decrease progressively;
(2) Peripheral blood inflammatory factors, such as IL-6 and CRP, increase progressively;
(3) Lactate increases progressively;
(4) Lung lesions develop rapidly in a short period.

2. *Children*

(1) Increased respiratory rate;
(2) Poor mental reaction and drowsiness;
(3) Lactate increases progressively;
(4) Imaging shows infiltration on both sides or multiple lobes, pleural effusion, or rapid progression of lesions in a short period;
(5) Infants under the age of 3 months who have either underlying diseases (congenital heart disease, bronchopulmonary dysplasia, respiratory tract deformity, abnormal hemoglobin, severe malnutrition, etc.) or immune deficiency or hypofunction (long-term use of immunosuppressants).

VIII. Differential Diagnosis

(1) The mild manifestations of NCP need to be distinguished from those of upper respiratory tract infections caused by other viruses.
(2) NCP is mainly distinguished from other known viral pneumonia and mycoplasma pneumonia infections such as influenza virus, adenovirus, and respiratory syncytial virus. For suspected cases, efforts should be made to use methods such as rapid antigen detection and multiplex PCR nucleic acid testing for the detection of common respiratory pathogens.
(3) NCP should also be distinguished from non-infectious diseases such as vasculitis, dermatomyositis, and organizing pneumonia.

IX. Case Finding and Reporting

Health professionals in medical institutions of all types and at all levels, upon discovering suspected cases that meet the definition, should immediately keep them in a separate room for quarantine and treatment. If the cases are still considered suspected after consultation by hospital experts or attending physicians, it should be reported directly online within 2 hours; samples should be subsequently collected for new coronavirus nucleic acid testing, and suspected cases should be safely transferred to the designated hospitals immediately. People who have been in close contact with confirmed patients are advised to report for new coronavirus pathogenic testing in a timely manner, even though common respiratory pathogens are tested positive.

If two nucleic acid tests, taken at least 24 hours apart, of an NCP suspected case are negative, and the NCP virus-specific IgM and IgG are negative seven days after onset, the suspect diagnosis can be ruled out.

X. Treatment

1. *Treatment venue determined by the severity of the disease*

(1) Suspected and confirmed cases should be quarantined and treated at designated hospitals with effective quarantine, protection, and prevention conditions in place. A suspected case should be treated in isolation in a single room. Confirmed cases can be treated in the same ward.

(2) Critical cases should be admitted to the ICU as soon as possible.

2. *General treatment*

(1) Rest in bed with strengthened support therapy and sufficient caloric intake; monitoring their water and electrolyte balance to maintain internal environment stability; closely monitoring vital signs and finger oxygen saturation.

(2) According to patients' conditions, monitoring blood routine results, urine routine result, C-reactive protein (CRP), biochemical indicators (liver enzyme, myocardial enzyme, renal function, etc.), coagulation function, arterial blood gas analysis, chest imaging, etc. Cytokines detection is recommended if necessary.

(3) Providing effective oxygen therapy in a timely manner, including nasal catheter and mask oxygenation and nasal high-flow oxygen

therapy. If possible, inhalation of mixed hydrogen and oxygen (H_2/O_2: 66.6%/33.3%) can be applied.

(4) Antiviral therapy: Alpha-interferon (5 million U or equivalent dose each time for adults, adding 2 ml of sterilized water, atomization inhalation twice daily), lopinavir/ritonavir (200 mg/50 mg per pill for adults, two pills each time, twice daily, no longer than ten days), Ribavirin (suggested to be used jointly with interferon or lopinavir/ritonavir, 500 mg each time for adults, two or three times of intravenous dripping daily, no longer than ten days), chloroquine phosphate (500 mg bid for 7 days for adults aged 18–65 with body weight over 50 kg; 500 mg bid for Days 1 & 2 and 500 mg QD for Days 3–7 for adults with body weight below 50 kg), or Arbidol (200 mg tid for adults, no longer than ten days).

Be aware of the adverse reactions, contraindications (for example, chloroquine is prohibited for patients with heart diseases), and possible drug-to-drug interactions. The efficacy of those drugs currently being used should be further evaluated in clinical use. Using three or more antiviral drugs at the same time is not recommended; if an intolerable toxic side effect occurs, the particular drug should be discontinued. The treatment of pregnant women should give due consideration to the number of gestational weeks, and the patients should be informed of choice of drugs having the least impact on the fetus, as well as whether pregnancy is being terminated before treatment.

(5) Antibiotic drug treatment: Irrational or inappropriate use of antibiotic drugs should be avoided, especially in combination with broad-spectrum antibiotics.

3. Treatment of severe and critical cases

3.1. Treatment principle

On the basis of symptomatic treatment, complications and secondary infections should be proactively prevented, underlying diseases should be treated, and organ function support should be provided in a timely manner.

3.2. Respiratory support

(1) Oxygen therapy: Patients with severe symptoms should receive nasal cannulas or masks for oxygen inhalation, and timely assessment of respiratory distress and/or hypoxemia should be performed.

(2) High-flow nasal catheter oxygenation or noninvasive mechanical ventilation: When respiratory distress and/or hypoxemia of the patient cannot be alleviated after receiving standard oxygen therapy, high-flow nasal cannula oxygen therapy or noninvasive ventilation can be considered. If conditions do not improve or even get worse within a short time (1–2 hours), tracheal intubation and invasive mechanical ventilation should be used in a timely manner.

(3) Invasive mechanical ventilation: Lung-protective ventilation strategy, namely, low tidal volume (6–8 ml/kg of ideal body weight) and low level of airway platform pressure (< 30 cmH$_2$O), should be used to perform mechanical ventilation to reduce ventilator-related lung injuries. While the airway platform pressure maintained ≤ 30 cmH$_2$O and high PEEP can be used to keep the airway warm and moist, avoid long sedation, and wake the patient early for lung rehabilitation. To prevent human–machine asynchronization, sedation and muscle relaxants should be used in a timely manner. Use closed sputum suction according to the airway secretion; if necessary, administer appropriate treatment based on bronchoscopy findings.

(4) Rescue therapy: Pulmonary re-tensioning is recommended for patients with severe ARDS. With sufficient human resources, prone position ventilation should be performed for more than 12 hours per day. If the outcome of prone position ventilation is poor, extracorporeal membrane oxygenation (ECMO) should be considered as soon as possible. Indications include the following: (1) When Fi02 > 90%, the oxygenation index is less than 80 mmHg for more than 3–4 hours; (2) For patients with only respiratory failure when the airway platform pressure ≥ 35 cmH$_2$O, VV-ECMO mode is preferred; if circulatory support is needed, VAECMO mode should be used. When underlying diseases are under control, and the cardiopulmonary function shows signs of recovery, withdrawal of ECMO can be tried.

3.3. *Circulatory support*

On the basis of adequate fluid resuscitation, efforts should be made to improve microcirculation by using vasoactive drugs, and closely monitoring changes in blood pressure, heart rate, and urine volume as well as lactate and base excess in arterial blood gas analysis. If necessary, use noninvasive or invasive hemodynamic monitors such as Doppler ultrasound, echocardiography, invasive blood pressure, or continuous cardiac output (PiCCO) monitoring. In the process of treatment, pay attention to the liquid balance strategy to avoid excessive or insufficient fluid intake.

If the heart rate suddenly increases more than 20% of the basic value or the decrease of blood pressure is more than 20% of the basic value with manifestations of poor skin perfusion and decreased urine volume, it should be closely observed whether the patient has septic shock, gastro-intestinal hemorrhage, or heart failure.

3.4. *Renal failure and renal replacement therapy*

Active efforts should be made to look for causes of renal function damage in critical cases such as low perfusion and drugs. For the treatment of patients with renal failure, the focus should be on the balance of body fluid, acid and base, and electrolyte balance, as well as on nutrition support, including nitrogen balance and the supplementation of energies and trace elements. For critical cases, continuous renal replacement therapy (CRRT) can be used. The indications include (1) hyperkalemia; (2) acidosis; (3) pulmonary edema or water overload; and (4) fluid management in multiple organ dysfunction.

3.5. *Convalescent plasma treatment*

It is suitable for patients with rapid disease progression, severe and critically ill patients. Usage and dosage should refer to the Protocol of Clinical Treatment with Convalescent Plasma for NCP Patients (2nd trial version).

3.6. *Blood purification treatment*

Blood purification system including plasma exchange, absorption, perfu-sion, and blood/plasma filtration can remove inflammatory factors and block "cytokine storm", so as to reduce the damage of inflammatory reac-tions to the body. It can be used for the treatment of severe and critical cases in the early and middle stages of the cytokine storm.

3.7. *Immunotherapy*

For patients with extensive lung lesions and severe cases who also show an increased level of IL-6 in laboratory testing, Tocilizumab can be used for treatment. The initial dose is 4–8 mg/kg, with the recommended dose of 400 mg diluted with 0.9% normal saline to 100 ml. The infusion should last for more than 1 hour. If the initial medication is not effective, one extra administration can be given 12 hours later (same dose as before). No more than two administrations should be given with the maximum single dose no more than 800 mg. Watch out for allergic reactions. The administration is forbidden for people with active infections such as tuberculosis.

3.8. *Other therapeutic measures*

For patients with progressive deterioration of oxygenation indicators, rapid progression of abnormalities in imaging, and excessive activation of the body's inflammatory response, glucocorticoids can be used in a short period of time (three to five days). It is recommended that the dose should not exceed the equivalent dose of methylprednisolone 1–2 mg/kg/day. Note that a larger dose of glucocorticoid delays the removal of coronavirus due to immunosuppressive effects. Xuebijing injection 100 ml/time can be administered twice a day intravenously. Intestinal microecological regulators can be used to maintain intestinal microecological balance and prevent secondary bacterial infections.

Severe and critical cases in children can be given an intravenous infusion of γ-globulin.

For pregnant severe and critical cases, pregnancy should be terminated, preferably with C-section.

Patients often suffer from anxiety and fear, and they should be supported by psychological counseling.

4. *Traditional Chinese medicine treatment*

Caused by the epidemic pathogenic factors, this disease falls in the category of pestilence in traditional Chinese medicine (TCM), According to the different local climate characteristics and individual state of illness and physical conditions, the following treatment protocol may vary. The use of over-pharmacopeia doses should follow the physician's instruction.

4.1. *During medical observation*

Clinical manifestation 1: Fatigue and gastrointestinal discomfort.

Recommended Chinese patent medicine: Huoxiang Zhengqi capsules (pills, liquid, or oral solution).

Clinical manifestation 2: Fatigue and fever.

Recommended Chinese patent medicine: Jinhua Qinggan granules, Lianhua Qingwen capsules (granules), Shufeng Jiedu capsules (granules), or Fangfeng Tongsheng pills (granules).

4.2. *During clinical treatment (confirmed cases)*

(1) Lung Cleansing & Detoxifying Decoction:

Scope of application: It is suitable for mild, moderate, and severe cases, and can be used with caution for critically ill patients with due consideration of their specific conditions.

Recommended prescription: Ephedra Herb (*Herba Ephedrae*) 9 g, Prepared Liquorice Root (*Glycyrrhizae radix et rhizoma praeparata cum melle*) 6 g, Bitter Apricot Seed (*Semen Armeniacae Amarum*) 9 g, Gypsum (*Gypsum Fibrosum*) 15–30 g (decocted first), Cassia Twig (*Ramulus Cinnamomi*) 9 g, Oriental Waterplantain Rhizome (*Rhizoma Alismatis*) 9 g, Agaric (*Polyporus*) 9 g, Largehead Atractylodes Rhizome (*Rhizoma Atractylodis Macrocephalae*) 9 g, Indian Buead (*Poria*) 15 g, Chinese Thorowax Root/Red Thorowax Root (*Radix Bupleuri*) 16 g, Baical Skullcap Root (*Radix Scutellariae*) 6 g, ginger processed Pinellia Tuber (*Pinelliae rhizoma praepatatum cum zingibere et alumine*) 9 g, fresh Ginger (*Zingiberis rhizoma recens*) 9 g, Tatarian Aster Root (*Radix Asteris*) 9 g, Common Coltsfoot Flower (*Flos Farfarae*) 9 g, Blackberrykiky Rhizome (*Rhizoma Belamcandae*) 9 g, Manchurian Wild ginger (*Herba Asari*) 6 g, Common Yam Rhizome (*Rhizoma Diosscoreae*) 12 g, Immature Bitter Orange (*Fructus Aurantii Immaturus*) 6 g, Tangerine Peel (*Pericarpium Citri Reticulatae*) 6 g, Cablin Potchouli Herb (*Herba Pogostemonis*) 9 g.

Suggested oral administration: Traditional Chinese medicine decoction pieces for decocting in water. One dose per day with each serving, both in the morning and evening (forty minutes after a meal), served in warm water, and three doses a course.

If conditions permit, the patient can take half a bowl of rice soup each time after taking medicine and can take up to one bowl if the patient has a dry tongue and is deficient in bodily fluids. (*Note*: If the patient does not have a fever, the amount of gypsum should be reduced. If there is a fever or even intense heat, the amount of gypsum can be increased.) If the symptoms persist despite certain improvements, then the second course of treatment should follow. If the patient has special conditions or other underlying diseases, the prescription of the second course of treatment can be modified based on the actual situation, and the medicine should be discontinued when the symptoms disappear.

Source of prescription: Notice on Recommending the Use of "Lung cleansing & detoxifying decoction" in Treatment of NCP by Integrated Traditional Chinese and Western Medicine by the Office of the State Administration of Traditional Chinese Medicine & the General Office of the National Health Commission (2022 No. 22).

(2) Mild cases:

(i)   Pattern of Cold-dampness Stagnating the Lung:

Clinical manifestations: Fever, fatigue, sore body, cough, expectoration, chest tightness, suffocation, loss of appetite, nausea, vomiting, and sticky stools. The tongue has a thin fat tooth mark or is faint red, and the coating is thick white or white greasy, and the pulse is soft or slippery.

Recommended prescription: Ephedra Herb 6 g, Gypsum 15 g (decocted first), Bitter Apricot Seed 9 g, Incised Notopterygium Rhizome/Forbes Notopterygium Rhizome (*Rhizoma Notopterygii*) 15 g, Pepperweed Seed/Tansymustard Seed (*Semen Lepidii/Semen Desurainiae*) 15 g, Cyrtomium Rhizome (*Rhizoma Cyrtomii*) 9 g, Earthworm (*Lumbricus*) 15 g, Paniculate Swallowwort Root (*Radix Cynanchi Paniculati*) 15 g, Cablin Potchouli Herb 15 g, Fortune Eupatorium Herb (*Herba Eupatorii*) 9 g, Chinese Atractylodes Rhizome (*Rhizoma Atractylodis*) 15 g, Poria from Yunnan of China 45 g, Largehead Atractylodes Rhizome 30 g, Jiao Sanxian [charred Hawthorn Fruit (*Crataegi Fructus*) 9 g, charred Medicated Leaven (*Massa medicate fermentata*) 9 g, and charred Malt (*Fructus Hordei Germinatus*) 9 g], Officinal Magnolia Bark (*Cortex Magnoliae Officinalis*) 15 g, Areca Seed (*Semen Arecae*) 9 g, Tsaoko Amomum Fruit (*Fructus Tsaoko*) 9 g, fresh Ginger 15 g.

Suggested oral administration: One dose daily, decocted in 600ml water, take it three times in the morning, noon, and evening before meals.

(ii) Pattern of Dampness-heat Accumulation in the Lung:

Clinical manifestations: Low or no fever, slight chills, fatigue, heavy head and body, muscle soreness, dry cough with little phlegm, sore throat, dry mouth with no desire to drink more, occasional chest tightness, no sweat or stagnated sweating, occasional vomiting and loss of appetite, and diarrhea or sticky stool. The tongue is reddish, and the coating is white, thick, and greasy or thin yellow, and the pulse is slippery or soft.

Recommended prescription: Areca Seed 10 g, Tsaoko Amomum Fruit 10 g, Officinal Magnolia Bark 10 g, Common Anemarrhena Rhizome (*Rhizoma Anemarrhena*) 10 g, Baical Skullcap Root 10 g, Chinese Thorowax Root 10 g, Red Paeony Root (*Radix Paeoniae Rubra*) 10 g, Weeping Forsythiae Capsule (*Fructus Forsythiae*) 15 g, Sweet Wormwood Herb (*Herba Artemisiae*) 10 g (decocted later), Chinese Atractylodes Rhizome 10 g, Indigowoad Leaf (*Folium Isatidis*) 10 g, Liquorice Root (*Radix Glycyrrhizae*) 5 g.

Suggested oral administration: One dose daily, decocted in 400-ml water divided into two times, one in the morning and one in the evening.

(3) Moderate cases:

(i) Pattern of Dampness-toxin Stagnating the Lung:

Clinical manifestations: Fever, cough with little sputum, or yellow sputum, suffocation, shortness of breath, bloating, and constipation. The tongue is dark red and fat; the coating is greasy or yellow, and the pulse is slippery or stringy.

Recommended prescription: Ephedra Herb 6 g, Bitter Apricot Seed 15 g, Gypsum 30 g (decocted first), Coix Seed (*Semen Coicis*) 30 g, Chinese Atractylodes Rhizome 10 g, Cablin Potchouli Herb 15 g, Sweet Wormwood Herb 12 g (decocted later), Giant Knotweed Rhizome (*Rhizoma Polygoni Cuspidati*) 20 g, European Verbena (*Herba Verbenae*) 30 g, Reed Rhizome (*Rhizoma Phragmitis*) 30 g, Pepperweed Seed 15 g, Pummelo Peel (*Exocarpium Citri Grandis*) 15 g, Liquorice Root 10 g.

Suggested oral administration: One dose daily, decocted in 400-ml water divided into two times, one in the morning and one in the evening.

(ii) Pattern of Cold-dampness Stagnating the Lung:

Clinical manifestations: Low fever, low body temperature, or no fever, dry cough with little sputum, lethargy, chest tightness, or nausea. The tongue is pale or red, the coating is white or greasy, and the pulse is soft.

Recommended prescription: Chinese Atractylodes Rhizome 15 g, Tangerine Peel 10 g, Officinal Magnolia Bark 10 g, Wrinkled Gianthyssop Herb 10 g, Tsaoko Amomum Fruit 6 g, Ephedra Herb 6 g, Incised Notopterygium Rhizome/Forbes Notopterygium Rhizome 10 g, fresh Ginger 10 g, Areca Seed 10 g.

Suggested oral administration: One dose daily, decocted in 400-ml water divided into two times, one in the morning and one in the evening.

(4) Severe cases:

(i) Pattern of Toxin Obstructing the Lung:

Clinical manifestations: Fever, flushing, cough with little yellowish and sticky phlegm, or blood in sputum, gasping, shortness of breath, lethargy, fatigue, dryness, stickiness and bitterness in mouth, nausea with no appetite, stagnated defecation, and short urination. Red tongue and greasy coating; slippery and rapid pulse.

Recommended prescription (Decoction of dampness-resolving and detoxification): Ephedra Herb 6 g, Bitter Apricot Seed 9 g, Gypsum 15 g (decocted first), Liquorice Root 3 g, Cablin Potchouli Herb 10 g (decocted later), Officinal Magnolia Bark 10 g, Chinese Atractylodes Rhizome 15 g, Tsaoko Amomum Fruit 10 g, Pinellia Tuber (*Rhizoma Pinelliae*) 9 g, Indian Buead 15 g, Rhubarb (*Radix et Rhizoma Rhei*) 5 g (decocted later), Mongolian Milkcetch Root (*Radix Astragali*) 10 g, Pepperweed Seed 10 g, Red Paeony Root 10 g.

Suggested oral administration: One or two doses daily, decocted in 100–200-ml water, take it 2–4 times, oral or nasal feeding.

(ii) Pattern of Flaring Heat in Qi and Ying Aspect:

Clinical manifestations: Intense fever, dysphoria and thirst, breathlessness, shortness of breath, blurred vision, delirious speech, or spotted rash, or vomiting blood, bleeding, or convulsions in the limbs. Tongue ridges have few or no moss with a rapid pulse, either sunken and fine or floating and large.

Recommended prescription: Gypsum 30–60 g (decocted first), Common Anemarrhena Rhizome 30 g, Common Anemarrhena Rhizome (*Radix Rehmanniae*) 30–60 g, Buffalo Horn (*Cornu Bubali*) 30 g (decocted first), Red Paeony Root 30 g, Figwort Root (*Radix Scrophulariae*) 30 g, Weeping Forsythiae Capsule 15 g, Tree Peony Bark (*Cortex Moutan*) 15 g, Golden Thread (*Rhizoma Coptidis*) 6 g, Common Lophatherum Herb (*Herba Lophatheri*) 12 g, Pepperweed Seed 15 g, Liquorice Root 6 g.

Suggested use: 1 dose per day, decoction, gypsum and buffalo horn decocted first, other pieces put in and decocted later, 100–200-ml each time, 2–4 times a day, orally or nasally.

Recommended Chinese patent medicines: Xiyanping injection, Xuebijing injection, Reduning injection, Tanreqing injection, or Xingnaojing injection. Among these drugs with similar efficacy, one can be selected according to individual conditions or two can be used concomitantly according to clinical symptoms. Traditional Chinese medicine injection can be used in combination with traditional Chinese medicine decoction.

(5) Critical cases:

Pattern of Inner Block and External Collapse:

Clinical manifestations: Dyspnea, gasping, or mechanical ventilation needed, coma, dysphoria, excessive sweating and cold limbs, dark purple tongue, thick or dry coating, and large and floating pulse.

Recommended prescription: Ginseng (*Radix Ginseng*) 15 g, Prepared Common Monkshood Branched Root (*Aconiti lateralis radix praeparata*)

10 g (decocted first), Common Macrocarpium Fruit (*Fructus Corni*) 15 g, delivered with Suhexiang Pill or Angong Niuhuang Pill.

For patients on mechanical ventilation with abdominal distention or constipation: 5–10 g of Rhubarb may be added. For patients with human–machine asynchronization: 5–10 g of Rhubarb and 5–10 g of Mirabilite (*Mirabilitum*) may be added while administering sedatives and muscle relaxants.

Recommended Chinese patent medicines: Xuebijing injection, Reduning injection, Tanreqing injection, Xingnaojing injection, Shenfu injection, Shengmai injection, or Shenmai injection. Among these drugs with similar efficacy, one can be selected according to individual conditions or two can be used concomitantly according to clinical symptoms. Traditional Chinese medicine injection can be used in combination with traditional Chinese medicine decoction.

Note: **Recommended usage of Chinese medicine injections for severe and critical cases**

The use of traditional Chinese medicine injections follows the principle of starting from a small dose and gradually adjusting the dosage according to the package insert. The recommended usage is as follows:

Viral infection or combined with mild bacterial infection: 0.9% sodium chloride injection 250 ml plus Xiyanping injection 100 mg bid, or 0.9% sodium chloride injection 250 ml plus Reduning injection 20 ml, or 0.9% sodium chloride injection 250 ml plus Tanreqing injection 40 ml bid.

High fever with disturbance of consciousness: 250 ml of 0.9% sodium chloride injection and 20 ml bid of Xingnaojing injection.

Systemic inflammatory response syndrome or/and multiple organ failure: 250 ml of 0.9% sodium chloride injection and 100 ml of Xuebijing injection.

Immunosuppression: 250 ml of 0.9% sodium chloride injection and 100 ml bid of Shenmai injection.

(6) Convalescent period:

(i) Pattern of Lung–spleen Qi Deficiency:

Clinical manifestations: Shortness of breath, lethargy, anorexia, nausea, abdominal fullness, and incomplete bowel movement with loose stool. The tongue is pale and greasy.

Recommended prescription: Pinellia Tuber 9 g, Tangerine Peel 10 g, Pilose Asiabell Root (*Radix Codonopsis*) 15 g, honey-fried Membranous Milkvetch Root/Mongolian Milkcetch Root 30 g, stir-fried Largehead Atractylodes Rhizome 10 g, Indian Buead 15 g, Cablin Potchouli Herb 10 g, Villous Amomum Fruit (*Fructus Amomi*) 6 g (decocted later), and Liquorice Root 6 g.

Suggested oral administration: 1 dose per day, decocted in 400-ml water divided into two times, one in the morning and one in the evening.

(ii) Pattern of Qi-yin Deficiency:

Clinical manifestations: Fatigue, shortness of breath, dry mouth, thirst, palpitations, sweating, poor appetite, low or no fever, dry cough with little sputum, dry tongue with little saliva, and fine or weak pulse.

Recommended prescription: Ladybell Root (*Radix Adenophorae*) 10 g, Coastal Glehnia Root (*Radix Glehniae*) 10 g, Dwarf Lilyturf Tuber (*Radix Ophiopogonis*) 15 g, American Ginseng (*Radix Panacis Quinquefolii*) 6 g, Chinese Magnoliavine Fruit (*Fructus Schisandrae*) 6 g, Gypsum 15 g (decocted first), Common Lophatherum Herb 10 g, Mulberry Leaf (*Folium Mori*) 10 g, Reed Rhizome 15 g, Danshen Root (*Radix Salviae Miltiorrhizae*) 15 g, Liquorice Root 6 g.

Suggested oral administration: 1 dose per day, decocted in 400-ml water divided into two times, one in the morning and one in the evening.

XI. Discharge Criteria and After-Discharge Considerations

1. *Discharge criteria*

(1) Body temperature is back to normal for more than three days;
(2) Respiratory symptoms improve markedly;
(3) Pulmonary imaging shows obvious absorption of inflammation;
(4) Nucleic acid tests negative twice consecutively on respiratory tract samples such as sputum and nasopharyngeal swabs (sampling interval being at least 24 hours).

Those who meet the above criteria can be discharged.

2. *After-discharge considerations*

(1) The designated hospitals should share patients' medical records with the primary healthcare institutions where the patients live and send the information of the discharged patients to the community and primary healthcare institutions where the patients reside.

(2) After discharge, it is recommended for patients to monitor their own health conditions and quarantine themselves at home wearing a mask for 14 days. It is recommended for them to live in a well-ventilated single room if possible, minimize close contact with family members, dine alone, practice hand hygiene, and avoid going out.

(3) It is recommended for the patients to return to the hospitals for follow-up and re-visit in the second and fourth week after discharge.

XII. Patients Transportation Principles

Patients should be transported in accordance with the *Work Protocol for Transfer of the Novel Coronavirus Pneumonia Patients* (*Trial Version*) issued by the National Health Commission.

XIII. Nosocomial Infection Prevention and Control

Measures to prevent and control nosocomial infection should be implemented in accordance with the requirements of the *Technical Guidelines for the Prevention and Control of Infection by the Novel Coronavirus in Medical Institutions* (*First Edition*) and *the Guidelines on the Usage of Common Medical Protective Equipment against Novel Coronavirus Infection* (*Trial Version*) formulated by the National Health Commission.

The General Office of National Health Commission

Office of State TCM Administration

Printed and distributed on March 3, 2020

Chapter 3

Rational Use of Chinese Patent Medicine

The World Health Organization (WHO) defines *rational use of medicines* if patients receive medications appropriate for their clinical needs, in doses that meet their own individual requirements, for an adequate period of time, and at the lowest cost to them and their community. In summary, the core components of rational use of medicines include safety, efficacy, economics, and appropriateness. The rational use of Chinese patent medicine also needs to conform to these core components. On top of that, the use of Chinese patent medicine is under the guidance of TCM theory. The essence of treatment based on pattern identification should be inherited to master the guiding principle of clinical use, ADRs/ADEs, precautions, and combination rules to ensure the safe and rational use of Chinese patent medicine.

Section 1: Guiding Principles for the Clinical Application of Chinese Patent Medicine

In June 2010, the State Administration of traditional Chinese medicine (SATCM) and the former Ministry of Health organized experts to formulate the guiding principles for clinical application of Chinese patent medicine (hereinafter referred to as the guiding principles), which aimed to improve the clinical efficacy of Chinese patent medicine, standardize the use of Chinese patent medicine, reduce the occurrence of adverse reactions of traditional Chinese medicine, reduce the medical costs of patients, and ensure the safety of the use of medication.

I. Safety of Chinese Patent Medicine

Chinese patent medicine has been used extensively throughout history. Chinese patent medicine is mostly safe when used rationally. Rational use includes accurate pattern diagnosis and appropriate selection of medicine, usage, dosage, treatment course, contraindications, concomitant medication, etc. To prevent adverse reactions of Chinese patent medicines, attention should be paid to the following aspects:

(1) Strengthen observation and monitoring of adverse reactions of traditional Chinese medicine during use of medicines, and improve the reporting system of adverse reactions of traditional Chinese medicine.

(2) Note the history of drug allergies. Patients with a history of drug allergies should be closely monitored after taking the drug. If there is an allergic reaction, the drug should be discontinued immediately and prompt measures be taken to prevent serious consequences.

(3) Medication use based on pattern diagnosis, a proper dose, and appropriate course of treatment should be followed. Especially for special groups, such as infants, the elderly, pregnant women, and patients with compromised organ function, more attention should be paid to the medication regimen.

(4) Be aware of drug-to-drug interactions (DDIs), especially when Chinese and Western medicines are used concomitantly.

(5) Monitoring safety indicators should be strengthened for patients who need long-term medication.

II. Basic Principles of Clinical Application of Chinese Patent Medicine

1. *Use medicines based on pattern diagnosis/syndrome differentiation*

According to the theory of traditional Chinese medicine, identify and analyze the pattern of the disease before determining the specific treatment for the disease and selecting the appropriate Chinese patent medicine.

2. *Medication selection based on both disease and pattern diagnosis*

Medication selection based on disease diagnosis is aimed at selecting the appropriate Chinese patent medicines based on the characteristics of the diseases that are either clearly defined in traditional Chinese medicine or with a clear diagnosis in Western medicine. When Chinese patent medicine is used clinically, the Chinese patent medicine can be selected through the combination of TCM pattern diagnosis/syndrome differentiation and TCM disease diagnosis or the combination of Western medicine disease diagnosis and TCM pattern diagnosis. Western medical diagnosis alone, however, cannot fulfill the rationale for the choice of Chinese patent medicine.

3. *Selection of dosage form*

The appropriate dosage form should be selected according to the physical condition of the patient, the severity of the disease, and the characteristics of various dosage forms.

4. *Determination of dosage*

For those with a definite dosage instruction, caution should be taken with overdose. For Chinese patent medicines with an expected dosage range, the dosage for the elderly should be within the lower limit.

5. *Rational administration route*

If it can be administered orally, do not use injection; if it can be administered intramuscularly, do not use intravenous injection or drip infusion.

6. *The use of Chinese medicine injection should also follow the below principles*

(1) The history of allergies should be inquired carefully before use, and those with allergies should use the medicines with caution.

(2) Strictly follow the instructions specified in the package insert; use drugs based on pattern diagnosis, and off-label use is prohibited.

(3) Chinese medicine injections should be used with the recommended dosage, requirements for preparations, dripping speed, and course of treatment specified in the package insert. Overdose, speedy dripping, and long-term use should be avoided.

(4) Traditional Chinese medicine injections should be used alone, and it is strictly forbidden to mix with other drugs. For long-term use, there must be a certain time interval between each treatment course.

(5) Strengthen drug monitoring. The patients' reaction should be closely observed during use, and the drug should be discontinued immediately if there are adverse reactions. Effective treatment measures should be taken if necessary. Cautions should be taken and monitoring should be strengthened for the elderly, children, people with liver and kidney dysfunction, and other patients who are using traditional Chinese medicine injections for the first time.

III. Principle for Combined Use

1. *Combined use of Chinese patent medicines*

(1) If it is a complex disease, whose treatment requires more than one Chinese patent medicine, multiple Chinese patent medicines can be used in combination.

(2) The combined application of multiple Chinese patent medicines should follow the principle of efficacy augmentation and toxicity reduction. In principle, Chinese patent medicines with the same or substantially the same functions should not be used simultaneously.

(3) Avoid repeated use for medicines with drastic potency or containing toxic ingredients.

(4) When combining medications, pay attention to the compatibility of components of Chinese patent medicine.

(5) For some diseases, internal medicine and external medicine can be used concomitantly.

The combined use of Chinese medicine injections should also follow the below principles:

(1) The combined use of two or more traditional Chinese medicine injections should follow the requirements of traditional Chinese medicine compatibility theory and the principle of efficacy augmentation and toxicity reduction.
(2) Be cautious in medication combinations. If combined use of medication is really needed, there should be an appropriate interval between TCM injections to avoid drug-to-drug interactions.
(3) When two or more traditional Chinese medicine injections are needed at the same time, mixing of these injections is strictly prohibited and they should be used separately. Unless otherwise specified, it is not advisable for two or more varieties of Chinese medicine injections to share the same vascular access at the same time.

2. Combined use of Chinese patent medicine and Western medicine

When formulating medication plans for specific diseases, consider the roles of Chinese and Western medicines to determine the dosage, time, and route of administration.

(1) If there is no clear contraindication between Chinese patent medicine and Western medicine, they can be used in combination. They should be used separately if they share the same route of administration.
(2) The combination of Chinese and Western medicines with similar side effects should be avoided, and the combination of Chinese and Western medicines with adverse interactions should also be avoided.

Combined use of TCM injections and western medicine injections should also follow the principles below:

(1) Be cautious. If the combined use is necessary, the selection of medication should be based on the disease/pattern diagnosis as well as principles with due consideration given to the possible drug-to-drug interaction. The number and dosage of the medications involved should be minimized. And, timely adjustments should be made based on clinical conditions.

(2) Different administration routes should be used when TCM injections and Western medicine injections are used in combination. If it is unavoidable to share the same administration route, they should be used at certain intervals. Careful consideration should be given to the interval and the possible drug-to-drug interactions. Mixing of medicine applications is prohibited.

IV. Principles of Use of Chinese Patent Medicine for Pregnant Women

(1) When pregnant women need to use medicine, they should choose Chinese patent medicine that does no harm to the fetus.
(2) Pregnant women should use Chinese patent medicines by oral administration. Chinese medicine injections should be used with caution. According to the therapeutic effect of Chinese patent medicine, the medication course for pregnant women should be as short as possible, and the dosage should be reduced or medication discontinued in time.
(3) Chinese patent medicines that may cause miscarriage or teratogenic effects on the fetus are prohibited in pregnancy. Most of these drugs contain toxic or violent ingredients, such as Arsenic (*Arsenicum*), Realgar (*Realgar*), Calomel (*Calomelas*), Blister Beetle (*Mylabris*), Toad Venom (*Venenum Bufonis*), Musk (*Moschus*), Nux Vomica (*Semen Strychni*), Aconite (*Aconiti Lateralis Radix Praeparaia*), Prepared Common Monkshood Branched Root (*Aconiti Lateralis Radix Praeparaia*), Ground Beetle (*Eupolyphaga seu Steleophaga*), Leech (*Hirudo*), Gadfly (*Tabanus*), Common Burreed Rhizome (*Rhizoma Sparganii*), Zedoary (*Rhizoma Curcumae*), Pokeberry Root (*Radix Phytolaccae*), Gansui Root (*Radix Kansui*), Knoxia Root (*Radix Knoxiae*), Lilac Daphne Flower Bud (*Flos Genkwa*), Pharbitis Seed (*Semen Pharbitidis*), and Croton Seed (*Semen Crotonis*).
(4) Medication that may cause abortion and other side effects should be used with great caution for pregnant women. This kind of medication mostly contains ingredients possessing the power of dredging channels and dispersing stasis such as the Peach Seed (*Semen Persicae*), Safflower (*Flos Carthami*), Twotooth Achyranthes Root (*Radix Achyranthis Bidentatae*), Cattail Pollen (*Pollen Typhae*), Trogopterus Dung (*Faeces Trogopterori*), Pangolin Scales (*Squama Manitis*), Cowherb Seed (*Semen Vaccariae*), Chinese Trumpetcreeper Flower

(*Flos Campsis*), Giant Knotweed Rhizome (*Rhizoma Polygoni Cuspidati*), Tamariskoid Spikemoss Herb (*Herba Selaginellae*), and Sanqi (*Radix Notoginseng*), or ingredients possessing the power of promoting qi flow and resolving the stagnation such as Immature Bitter Orange (*Fructus Aurantii Immaturus*), Rhubarb, Mirabilite (*Mirabilitum*), Senna Leaf (*Folium Sennae*), Chinese Dwarf Cherry Seed/Dwarf Flowering Cherry Seed/Longstalk Peach Seed and (*SemenPruni*); or Dried Ginger (*Rhizoma Zingiberis*), Cassia Bark (*Cortex Cinnamomi*), etc.; Cluster Mallow Fruit (*Fructus Malvae Vertillatae*), Lilac Pink Herb (*Herba Dianthi*), Akebia Stem (*Caulis Akebiae*), Uniflower Swisscentaury Root (*Radix Rhapontici*), etc.

V. Principles for the Use of Chinese Patent Medicine Among Children

(1) The physiological particularities of children deserve special attention when using Chinese patent medicines. According to the physiological characteristics of children at different ages, appropriate drugs and applications should be considered. Both effectiveness and safety should be taken into account when determining the dosage of Chinese patent medicines for children.

(2) It is advisable to use Chinese patent medicines specifically developed for children. In general, the dosage of Chinese patent medicines for children at different ages/weights is listed in the package insert. Follow the pre-specified appropriate dosage accordingly.

(3) If the Chinese patent medicine used is not for children only, dosage determination should be made on account of the specific conditions to ensure effectiveness and safety. The corresponding dosage should be determined according to the children's age and weight. In general, 1/4 adult dose is recommended for children within three years of age; 1/3 adult dose is recommended for children 3–5 years of age; 1/2 adult dose is recommended for children 5–10 years of age, and the adult dose can be considered for children 10 years of age.

(4) When using Chinese patent medicines containing highly toxic ingredients, or Chinese patent medicines containing special ingredients toxic for children and infants, the risks/benefits should be carefully weighed. Generally, such medicines should not be considered for clinical use unless it is absolutely necessitated.

(5) It is not recommended for children to use varied types of Chinese patent medicines. Oral and external administration should be the first choice, and Chinese medicine injections should be used with caution.

(6) According to the therapeutic effect, the medication course of children should be shortened in minimum, and the dosage should be reduced or medication discontinued in time.

Section 2: Contraindications in the Use of Chinese Patent Medicine

In the use of Chinese patent medicine, in order to ensure the curative effect and avoid adverse effects, there are some contraindications in the clinical application of Chinese patent medicine. The contraindications in the use of Chinese patent medicine can be summarized as the following four situations:

I. Contraindicated Patterns/Syndromes

Treatment based on pattern diagnosis/syndrome differentiation is the primary principle to guide the use of Chinese patent medicine. For the same disease, different medicines should be used for different patterns identified. Therefore, the clinical application of Chinese patent medicine should strictly follow the contraindications of syndromes.

For example, for those who suffer from headache and cough caused by exposure to exogenous cold and fever, they should use Ganmaoqing Capsule with caution as it is a pungent-cool exterior-releasing medicine; those who suffer from blood stasis and coma due to cold closure should be forbidden to use Angong Niuhuang Pill; and those who are in the middle of menstruation or those who have not completely stopped bleeding following intracranial hemorrhage should be forbidden to use Xinnao Shutong Capsule, etc.

II. Contraindicated Combination (Incompatibility)

Incompatibility mainly refers to that the risks of producing toxicity, serious side effects or reducing efficacy when some medicines are used in combination with other herbs in different prescriptions. And, these herbs are thus forbidden to use in combination. In the long history of medical practice, traditional Chinese medicine has formed a set of complete compatibility methods as well as strict compatibility contraindications, which have been followed by the majority of medical professionals, such as "eighteen clashes" and "nineteen incompatibilities".

Although there are still some controversies, it is necessary to remain cautious before the mechanism is fully clarified. The Pharmacopoeia of the People's Republic of China (2015 edition) still lists "eighteen clashes" and "nineteen incompatibilities" as the compatibility contraindications; therefore, the combined use of these herbs should be avoided as much as possible. The two principles of "eighteen clashes" and "nineteen incompatibilities" should always be given due consideration when it comes to the combined use of different Chinese patent medicines, or the combined use of Chinese patent medicines and decoction.

In the clinical application of Chinese patent medicine, it is necessary to strictly follow the incompatibility rules of medicines, pay attention to the positive and negative effects of the combination of different drugs, and apply them properly in order to improve the clinical therapeutic effect.

III. Contraindications During Pregnancy

Some traditional Chinese medicines that have strong effects, such as breaking blood stasis to promote menstruation, promoting qi movement and removing obstruction, removing water retention by purgation, and purging and discharging with pungent and heat properties may lead to serious consequences of abortion or fetal damage. All the Chinese patent medicines that affect the normal development of the fetus and cause adverse reactions in pregnant women are contraindicated during pregnancy. Drugs that are prohibited must not be taken; drugs that are contraindicated in principle cannot be used; and drugs that can be used with caution should be used carefully according to the specific circumstances of pregnant women.

Maixuekang capsules, Shuxuetong injection, Niuhuang Jiedu tablets, Weitong Ning tablets, Xiao Huo Luo pills, and other Chinese patent medicines are all prohibited for pregnant women; Xiaoshuan Tongluo tablets, Huoxue Jiedu pills, Sanqi tablets, Babaodan capsules, and Shanzha Huazhi Pills are contraindicated for pregnant women; and Xuesaitong Granules, Lidan Tablets, Sanhuang Tablets, Niuhuang Shangqing Pills, Chuanxiong Chatiaowan, etc., should be used with caution for pregnant women.

IV. Contraindications in Diet

The use of Chinese patent medicines requires abstaining from certain food. For example, during the period of taking Chinese patent medicines, it is generally required to abstain from raw, cold, greasy, irritating and heavy foods that are not easy to digest. Heat pattern requires abstaining from spicy and greasy food; cold pattern requires abstaining from raw and cold food; the occurrence of edema requires abstaining from food with a very high salt content; acid reflux requires abstaining from vinegar; beginning of measles requires abstaining from greasy and sour food; insomnia requires abstaining from strong tea; and some skin diseases and sore boils require abstaining from fish, shrimp, mutton, etc.

In addition to the general contraindications, there are some special contraindications: Chenxiang Huazhi pills should not be taken concomitantly with medicine containing ginseng (*Radix Ginseng*); raw radish should not be taken when taking Chinese patent medicine containing ginseng and American ginseng (*Radix Panacis Quinquefolii*); when taking Jiawei Xiaoyao Pills, avoid fatigue and anger; and when suffering from cold, stop taking tonics, such as Guiling Paste and Dingkun Pellet.

Section 3: Adverse Reactions and Adverse Events of Chinese Patent Medicine

In recent years, with the development of social economy and the continuous progress of the pharmaceutical technology of Chinese patent medicine, the number of new varieties and new dosage forms of Chinese patent medicine has been increasing, which provides a much wider range of selection for clinical practitioners, and also contributes to the increasingly widespread application of Chinese patent medicine.

Meanwhile, there are an increasing number of reports about the adverse reactions of Chinese patent medicine. Adverse Drug Reaction (ADR) refers to any adverse, undesired, or unintended response to a legitimate therapeutic agent, which may be expected or unexpected, and may occur at normal dosages used for the prophylaxis, diagnosis, or therapy of disease, or for modifying physiologic function. ADRs do not include therapeutic failures, poisoning, and accidental or intentional overdoses. An adverse drug event (ADE) is an injury resulting from medical intervention related to a drug. ADEs include medication errors, adverse drug reactions, allergic reactions, and overdoses; they may not be directly associated with the medicines.

According to the 2017 ADR report released by the State Food and drug administration, in 2017, the number of ADR/AE reports in China reached 1.429 million, of which chemical drugs accounted for 82.8%, traditional Chinese medicine accounted for 16.1%, and biological products accounted for 1.1%. In 2017, the national ADR monitoring network received 592,000 ADR/AE reports, including 55,000 serious adverse events reports, accounting for 9.2%. Chemical and biological products accounted for 84.1% and another 15.9% went to Chinese patent medicine.

I. Factors Causing ADRs/ADEs of Chinese Patent Medicine

There are many causes for the occurrence of adverse reactions/adverse events in Chinese patent medicines, which can be summed up in the following three aspects: medicines, patients, and clinical use.

1. Medicines

1.1. The ingredients of traditional Chinese medicines

The occurrence of ADRs/ADEs of traditional Chinese medicine is often directly related to its chemical ingredients. For example, strychnine in nux vomica (*Semen Strychni*) and triptolide in Common Threewingnut Root (*Tripterygium wilfordii*) are the sources of toxicity, and deserve special caution.

1.2. Misuse and Misapplication

Some Chinese patent medicines sharing the same name, yet containing different herbs, are likely to lead to ADRs/ADEs or even poisoning if misused or misapplied clinically. For example, two different formulas sharing the same name of Jiming powder were recorded in two books: one titled *Treatise on Diseases, Patterns, and Formulas Related to the Unification of the Three Etiologies* (*San Yin Ji Yi Bing Zheng Fang Lun*) of the Song Dynasty and another one titled *Criterion of Pattern and Treatment for Pediatrics* (Zheng Zhi Zhun Shen Er Ke) of the Ming Dynasty. These two formulas have totally different components and therapeutic effects.

Huoxiang Zhengqi liquid and Huoxiang Zhengqi pill seem to be just different dosage forms of the same variety, but in fact, the composition of the two Chinese patent medicines is different. There is ethanol in Huoxiang Zhengqi liquid, which should be used with great caution.

1.3. Quality of medicinal substances

The ingredients and quality of Chinese patent medicine may differ depending on the variety, place of origin, harvest season, medicinal parts, and storage and transportation conditions. Therefore, the ingredients in different batches of the same traditional Chinese medicine may vary greatly. The pollution of the growth environment and the use of pesticides can increase the content of heavy metals (lead, arsenic, mercury, cadmium, etc.) and toxic ingredients in the medicine. In addition, improper storage and transportation methods are likely to give rise to propagation of bacteria and fungi in the medicinal materials, even leading to deterioration. These conditions can be the causes of adverse reactions/adverse events.

1.4. *Improper processing or manufacturing*

The processing and manufacturing technology of traditional Chinese medicine directly affects its efficacy. Some traditional Chinese medicine containing toxic ingredients or having a strong power can be rid of its toxicity and possible adverse effects through reasonable and correct processing; on the contrary, the improper processing and preparation of traditional Chinese medicine will lead to the occurrence of ADRs/ADEs. For example, in the case of improper processing of aconite, if it is also administered in a regular dose, it may lead to toxic reactions.

1.5. *Non-standard package insert*

It is necessary to strictly follow the instructions on the package insert when using the medicine, but sometimes the instructions of Chinese patent medicine are not standardized or complete. Many just state that no adverse reactions have been found, and the contraindications are not clear. These statements may easily mislead patients into misuse, thus increasing the risks of ADRs/ADEs.

2. Patients

2.1. *Special populations*

The elderly and children are more sensitive to drug toxicity because of their poor tolerance. Women, on the contrary, have poor tolerance to toxic drugs during menstruation, pregnancy, lactation, and menopause. In addition, patients with liver and kidney dysfunction are also prone to adverse drug reactions/events.

2.2. *Idiosyncrasy*

Individuals differ in genetics, metabolism, enzyme system, lifestyle, and hobbies. Therefore, different individuals may have different biological reactions to the same dose of the same drug, which shows that different individuals also have individual differences in terms of ADRs/ADEs of traditional Chinese medicine.

3. Clinical use

3.1. Inaccurate pattern diagnosis

Treatment based on pattern identification is the essence of traditional Chinese medicine, and inaccurate pattern diagnosis goes against this principle and tends to cause ADRs/ADEs. For example, in some comprehensive hospitals, some doctors may have prescribed Chinese patent medicine based on an oversimplified connection between the name of the Chinese patent medicine and the name of the disease. This malpractice has led to a large number of ADRs/ADEs of Chinese patent medicine.

Furthermore, many traditional Chinese medicines have become easily available OTC in drugstores and pharmacies in recent years. Quite a number of patients may go there, buy, and take traditional Chinese medicine on their own initiative without knowing the principle of treatment based on pattern identification of traditional Chinese medicine, leading to increased reports of ADRs/ADEs of Chinese patent medicine.

3.2. Overdose and prolonged use

There are some misconceptions that side effects of traditional Chinese medicine are mild, and the dosage range is flexible. Some patients tend to increase dosage or prolong use without consulting professionals, resulting in possible accumulation of toxicity, which can easily lead to damage of the liver and kidney. The excessive or long-term use of Chinese patent medicines containing Common Threewingnut Root (*Radix Tripterygii Wilfordii*) can cause liver and kidney impairment. The improper use of Chinese patent medicines containing toad venom (*bufonis venenum*) will injure the heart and cause arrhythmia. Chinese patent medicines containing strychnine can cause nervous system damage if overdosed. Chinese patent medicines containing Nux Vomica (*Semen Strychni*), Manchurian Dutchmanspipe Stem (*Caulis aristolochiae manshuriensis*), and Dutchmanspipe Fruit (*Fructus Aristolochiae*) cause nephrotoxicity. Prolonged use of some traditional Chinese medicine will lead to addiction, especially some Chinese patent medicines containing ephedrine, poppy shell, or codeine.

3.3. *Improper combination*

Chinese medicinal herbs are used in combination in one single prescription, so most of the Chinese patent medicines consist of a variety of herbs. In ancient times, there were records of compatibility contraindications of "eighteen clashes" and "nineteen incompatibilities". In addition to the ADRs/ADEs caused by the improper combination of different varieties of traditional Chinese medicine, adverse reactions/events caused by the improper combination of traditional Chinese medicine and Western medicine are also not uncommon. The rational combination of Chinese and Western medicine can supplement each other and enhance efficacy. If the combination is not proper, it can play an antagonistic role, resulting in the decrease of the efficacy and even lead to ADRs/ADEs.

II. Management of ADRs/ADEs of Chinese Patent Medicines

In order to maximize the efficacy of Chinese patent medicine and minimize the occurrence of ADRs/ADEs, it is necessary to use Chinese patent medicine properly.

1. *Right medicines for the right pattern*

Although the components of Chinese patent medicine are fixed, modification of certain ingredients is not as flexible as that of decoction. However, treatment based on pattern diagnosis/syndrome differentiation should also be the overriding premise in the use of traditional Chinese medicine. An incorrect diagnosis naturally leads to the wrong prescriptions. The use of "hot medicine" for "heat pattern" and "cold medicine" for "cold pattern" is no different from adding fuel to the untoward fire, thus aggravating the disease condition. Chinese patent medicine is developed for the treatment of various disease patterns, each of which has its own indications. It must be properly selected according to the syndrome types and symptoms of patients.

2. *Knowing about the Chinese patent medicine before use*

Knowing about the Chinese patent medicine before use means to learn about the main composition, usage, dosage, and pros and cons of compatibility of Chinese patent medicine. Such knowledge is the necessary prerequisite for the rational use of Chinese patent medicine. A comprehensive and accurate understanding of the composition and function of Chinese patent medicine can be obtained from the national drug standard and the package insert of Chinese patent medicine, including all key elements such as drug name, main ingredients, functions and indications, usage and dosage, adverse reactions, contraindications, precautions, expiry date, and approval number. These are authoritative and legal sources of information for understanding the actions and use of drugs. The administration of Chinese patent medicine is clearly specified in the drug standard and package insert. The rational use of Chinese patent medicine must be in strict accordance with the instructions, including the correct route of administration, duration, and other parameters of administration. The contraindications and precautions in the instructions must be strictly observed.

3. *Treatment in accordance with season, region, and patient*

The selection of Chinese patent medicine should differ according to the patients' gender, age, and physical condition, seasonal changes, and regional differences.

To start with, each gender has its own physiological characteristics such as female patients having different stages of menstruation, pregnancy, postpartum, etc.

Age is another factor. If the age of patient is different, the physiological functions and pathological changes are also different. The elderly tend to be deficient in kidney qi, qi, and blood, and hypoactive in organ functions; children have vigorous physiological function, yet with a lack of qi and blood and not fully developed organs. To treat different patients, we should use drugs flexibly according to these physiological and pathological characteristics.

In the aspect of physique, because of the differences in each individual's congenital constitution and lifestyles, the physical conditions also differ from one to another. Even if people are suffering from the same disease, the treatment and usage of medicine may differ. The selection of Chinese patent medicines should also be adjusted based on the seasonal and regional differences.

4. *Rational concomitant medications*

In order to enhance the efficacy and reduce the side effects while giving full consideration to clinical complex conditions of different patients, it is often necessary to use different Chinese patent medicines concomitantly or Chinese patent medicine together with Western medicine. In the process of concomitant medication, it is necessary to fully understand the compatibility and application principles of Chinese patent medicine from relevant reports, so as to avoid the occurrence of ADRs/ADEs.

5. *Proper dosage & dosage forms*

Due to different dosage forms or routes of administration, the same medicine may show different effects in terms of efficacy, indication range, and safety. Drug dosage is an important factor in the occurrence of biological effects of drugs. Different doses of drugs have different characteristics in absorption, distribution, metabolism, and excretion, thus affecting the drug efficacy. Reasonable drug dosage means not only the maximization of its efficacy but also the minimization of the incidence of adverse ADRs/ADEs.

In addition, it is essential to improve the quality of Chinese patent medicine by giving full play to the active role of the national ADRs/ADEs monitoring network and strengthening the exchange and research of relevant information; improving the formulation of regulatory laws and regulations on ADRs/ADEs; and attaching greater importance to the research of ADRs/ADEs. At the same time, it is necessary to further promote the reevaluation of Chinese patent medicine after it is put into market for sale by re-recognizing the safety, effectiveness, and economic value of Chinese patent medicine so as to further improve the safety of the application of Chinese patent medicine, promote the rational use of drugs, and improve the clinical efficacy of Chinese patent medicine.

Chapter 4

Guidance on Rational Application of Chinese Patent Medicine during Medical Observation Period

The *Diagnosis and Treatment Protocol for Novel Coronavirus Pneumonia* (Trial Version 7), issued by the National Health Commission and State Administration of Traditional Chinese Medicine, recommends the use of following Chinese Patent Medicines during the medical observation period: Huoxiang Zhengqi Capsule (pill, water, oral liquid), Jinhua Qinggan Granule, Lianhua Qingwen Capsule (granule), and Shufeng Jiedu Capsule.

Section 1: Huoxiang Zhengqi Capsule (see Table 3) (Pill, Water, Oral Liquid)

Boxed Warning:

> **This medicine contains Pinellia Tuber (*Rhizoma Pinelliae*), Liquorice Root (*Radix Glycyrrhizae*); tincture with ethanol as an excipient; be wary of compatibility issues. This product is contraindicated for allergic individuals and those who are allergic to this product.**

【Actions】Releasing exterior and resolving dampness, regulating qi, and harmonizing stomach.

【Indications】Common cold caused by exogenous wind-cold, endogenous dampness or summer heat dampness with the symptoms of headache and lethargy, chest and gastric fullness, epigastric distending pain, vomiting and diarrhea, and gastrointestinal colds. It is also used for gastrointestinal disorders such as functional dyspepsia, post-operative bowel distension, irritable bowel syndrome, acute gastroenteritis, diabetic diarrhea, viral enteritis, stomach or duodenal ulcers, and acute and chronic colitis.

Different dosage forms of Huoxiang Zheng qi have different ingredients, quality specifications, descriptions, administration and dosage, and strengths. See Table 1 for details.

【Side Effects】

Note: Based on the summary of observed clinical adverse events, this section aims to present a comprehensive profile of all possible safety events of this product, and does not include specific data about the incidence, severity, and scope of adverse events or adverse reactions (ADEs/ADRs).

The odds of adverse reactions are higher due to the use of ethanol as an excipient in the Huoxiang Zhengqi water. According to the literature, it has been reported that Huoxiang Zhengqi water can cause drug rash, purpura, allergic asthma, drunken allergy, anaphylactic shock and other allergic reactions, intestinal obstruction, upper gastrointestinal bleeding, pediatric hypoglycemia, pediatric convulsions, and disulfiram-like reactions.

Table 1. Comparison of Huoxiang Zhengqi drugs of different formulations.

	Huoxiang Zhengqi capsule	Huoxiang Zhengqi pill	Huoxiang Zhengqi water	Huoxiang Zhengqi oral liquid
Ingredients	Cabin Potchouli Herb (*Herba Pogostemonis*), Perilla Leaf (*Folium Perillae*), Dahurian Angelica Root (*Radix Angelicae Dahuricae*), Largehead Atractylodes Rhizome (*Rhizoma Atractylodis Macrocephalae*), Tangerine Peel (*Pericarpium Citri Reticulatae*), processed Pinellia Tuber (*Rhizoma Pinelliae Preparatum*), ginger processed Officinal Magnolia Bark (*Cortex Magnoliae Officinalis*), Indian Bread (*Poria*), Platycodon Root (*Radix Platycodi*), Liquorice Root (*Radix Glycyrrhizae*), Areca Peel (*Pericarpium Arecae*), Chinese Date (*Fructus Jujubae*), Fresh Ginger (*Rhizoma Zingiberis Recens*). Excipient is starch	Concentrated pill and water pill: same as Huoxiang Zhengqi capsule; Dropping pill: same as Huoxiang Zhengqi Oral Liquid	Swordlike Atractylodes Rhizome (*Rhizoma Atractylodis*), Tangerine Peel, ginger processed officinal Magnolia Bark, Dahurian Angelica Root, Indian Bread, Areca Peel, Pinellia Tuber, Extractum Glycyrrhizae, oil of Cablin Potchouli Herb, oil of Perilla Leaf. Excipient is ethanol	Swordlike Atractylodes Rhizome (*Rhizoma Atractylodis*), Tangerine Peel, ginger processed officinal Magnolia Bark, Dahurian Angelica Root, Indian Bread, Areca Peel, Pinellia Tuber, Extractum Glycyrrhizae, oil of Cablin Potchouli Herb, oil of Perilla Leaf
Quality Specification	National Drug Standards: WS3-B-2266-96-2002	Concentrated pill: "National Drug Standards of the Ministry of Health" the seventh volume of Chinese traditional medicine prescription WS3-B-1465-93; Water pill: Pharmacopoeia of the People's Republic of China (1990 edition one) Dropping pill: Pharmacopoeia of the People's Republic of China (2015 edition one)	Pharmacopoeia of the People's Republic of China (2015 edition one)	Pharmacopoeia of the People's Republic of China (2015 edition one)

(*Continued*)

Table 1. (*Continued*)

	Huoxiang Zhengqi capsule	Huoxiang Zhengqi pill	Huoxiang Zhengqi water	Huoxiang Zhengqi oral liquid
Description	The contents are red-brown particles, sweet and slightly bitter	Concentrated pill: dark brown, fragrant, sweet, slightly bitter; Water pill: greenish yellow to brownish yellow, fragrant, sweet, slightly bitter; Dropping pill: yellow-brown to brown after removing the coating, aroma, spicy, slightly sweet, bitter	Dark brown clear liquid (slightly precipitated during storage), spicy and bitter	brown clear liquid, spicy and slightly sweet
Administration and Dosage	Oral, 4 capsules at a time, 2 times a day	Concentrated pill: Oral, 8 pills at a time, 3 times a day; Water pill: oral, 6 g once, twice a day; Dropping pill: Oral, 1–2 sachets a time, 2 times a day, 5–10 ml each time, 2 times a day, shake well when used	Oral, 5 ~ 10 ml once, twice a day, shake well when used	Oral, 5 ~ 10 ml once, twice a day, shake well when used
Strengths	0.3 g/grain	Concentrated pill: every 8 pills is equivalent to 3 g of original medicine; Water pill: 6 g/bag; Dropping pill: 2.6 g/bag	10 ml/stick	10 ml/stick

The clinical manifestations of disulfiram-like reactions are chest tightness, shortness of breath, laryngeal edema, cyanosis, dyspnea, increased heart rate, decreased blood pressure, facial flushing, decreased vision, headache, insomnia, drowsiness, hallucinations, and even anaphylactic shock.

I. Drug–Drug Interactions Among Concomitant Medications

1. *Concomitant medications*

1.1. *The "eighteen clashes" in the combined use of Chinese herbal medicine*

This product contains Pinellia Tuber, which clashes with Aconitum, [including Prepared Common Monkshood Daughter Root (*Radix Aconiti Lateralis Preparata*), Common Monkshood Mother Root (*Radix Aconiti*), and Kusnezoff Monkshood Root (*Radix Aconiti Kusnezoffii*)]; and Liquorice Root, which is contraindicated in combination with Seaweed (*Sargassum*), Peking euphorbia root (*Radix Euphorbiae Pekinensis*), Lilac Daphne Flower Bud (*Flos Genkwa*), and Gansui Root (*Radix Kansui*); none of the above can be taken together.

1.2. *Combined use of Western medicines*

(1) Gastrointestinal reactions of other medicines:

The liquorice root contained in this product can interact with aspirin and cause an exacerbation of digestive tract disorders. The irritating effect of aspirin on the gastric mucosa and the glucocorticoid-like effect of liquorice root lead to the increase of gastric acid secretion, reduction of gastric mucus secretion, and reduction of the resistance of the gastrointestinal tract, thus inducing or aggravating gastric and duodenal ulcers.

Aspirin also has an anticoagulant effect, so it is often not easy to control once there is bleeding. The most common clinical adverse reactions of antipyretic analgesics are the gastrointestinal reaction caused by damage to the gastrointestinal mucosa. Alcohol has a damaging effect on the gastric mucosal barrier, so it can aggravate gastrointestinal reactions, such as gastritis, gastric ulcer, or the original ulcer, or even bleeding and perforation. In addition, if patients take alcoholic products while taking cimetidine for the treatment of ulcer disease, they are prone to toxic reactions because the drug inhibits alcohol metabolism in addition to the consequence that it is difficult to make the ulcer heal.

The non-steroidal anti-inflammatory drug aspirin can increase the irritation of the digestive tract when it is taken in large doses together with alcoholic products, which can easily cause gastric mucosal lesions or relapse ulcers, leading to gastrointestinal bleeding.

(2) Disulfiram-like reactions:

Huoxiang Zhengqi water contains alcohol, which is likely to lead to disulfiram-like reactions and exacerbate alcoholism. If alcoholic drinks are ingested while cephalosporins (such as cefoperazone, cefoperazone sulbactam, ceftriaxone, cefazolin, cefmetazole, cefminol, moxalactam, cefmenoxime, and cefamandole), nitiomidazoles (metronidazole, tinidazole, ornidazole, and secnidazole), other antimicrobial drugs (such as furazolidone, chloramphenicol, ketoconazole, and griseofulvin), tolbutamide, glibenclamide, phenformin, and other drugs are taken at the same time, it will lead to accumulation of acetaldehyde in the body and trigger a poisoning reaction, which is called disulfiram-like reaction. Therefore, alcohol should not be taken with the above drugs.

(3) Synergistic effects on some medicines:

Alcohol has obvious synergistic effects on calcium channel blockers, monoamine oxidase inhibitors, metoclopramide, hydrochlorothiazide, reserpine, acetaminophen, and central inhibitors such as phenobarbital, chlordiazepoxide, methaqualone, chloral hydrate, diazepam, chlorpromazine, fluphenazine, doxepin, chlorpheniramine, and tricyclic antidepressants in Huoxiang Zhengqi water. The above drugs can increase the inhibitory effect on the central nervous system by preventing the oxidation of alcohol, leading to the lethal dose reduction. Therefore, alcohol-containing drugs should not be combined with central inhibitor drugs.

(4) Effects on metabolism of other drugs:

Alcohol in Huoxiang Zhengqi water is a liver drug enzyme inducer, which can enhance the activity of liver drug enzymes, accelerate drug metabolism, and reduce drug efficacy. If a patient with epilepsy drinks alcohol while taking phenytoin, he cannot effectively control the seizures, which is the result of alcohol's accelerated metabolism of phenytoin by liver drug enzyme induction. Alcohol can also accelerate the metabolism of tolbutamide through the induction of liver drug enzymes.

Alcohol and insulin, oral hypoglycemic drugs, are synergistic in function, because alcohol and hypoglycemic drugs have the effect of inhibiting gluconeogenesis; synergy between the two will cause severe hypoglycemia and neuropathy. Alcohol interferes with the absorption and storage of vitamin A, B vitamins, vitamin D, folic acid and calcium, magnesium, zinc, sodium, phosphorus, and other trace elements. Clinically, night blindness, dermatitis, loss of appetite, anepithymia, arrhythmia, and limb numbness, mental and memory loss, and other symptoms can occur. The combination of ethanol and methotrexate can interfere with the synthesis of choline and increase the toxicity to the liver, resulting in increased transaminases.

(5) Intensify the effect of other drugs to dilate blood vessels and weaken myocardial contractility:

Coronary heart disease patients taking nitrate drugs or patients taking antihypertensive drugs or diuretics may suffer excessive blood vessel dilation, postural hypotension, dizziness, weakness, etc., even cardiovascular collapse for some severe cases if they take alcohol at the same time.

(6) Weakening the efficacy of drugs:

Metoclopramide should not be taken while taking Huoxiang Zhengqi. Although both have anti-emetic functions, the mechanisms of their actions are different. Metoclopramide enhances the peristalsis of the stomach and esophagus and strengthens the ability to clear the contents of the esophagus to promote the emptying of the stomach contents and to promote the relaxation of the pylorus, duodenum, and upper jejunum, contributing to the coordination of the functions of the stomach, body, and upper intestine to achieve the purpose of stopping vomiting. Huoxiang Zhengqi preparations stop vomiting by inhibiting the activity of the gastrointestinal smooth muscle. Therefore, the simultaneous use of the two can produce pharmacological antagonism, which greatly reduces the efficacy of metoclopramide or reduces the efficacy of both.

2. Recommendations

Huoxiang Zhengqi water contains alcohol, liquorice root, Pinellia Tuber, etc. So, the herbs of "eighteen clashes" in traditional Chinese medicine and the compatibility in the combined use with alcohol and glucocorticoid-like ingredients deserve special attention. Concomitant medications with the abovementioned drugs should be avoided to ensure safe and effective medication.

II. Pharmacological Action

1. *Antispasmodic and analgesic effects*

It has an obvious inhibitory effect on the isolated duodenum of rabbits, and can resist intestinal spasm caused by cholinomimetic drugs. It is similar to the effect of atropine against intestinal spasm caused by salicylic acid and physostigmine. It has an obvious analgesic effect on visceral body reflex pain caused by acetic acid stimulating intestinal serosa or mesentery.

2. *Immunity-enhancing effects*

On mice with diarrhea induced by magnesium sulfate after treatment with Huoxiang Zhengqi pill, the 3H-TdR index of the peripheral blood lymphocyte infiltration increased, suggesting that the drug can improve the immune function of mice and promote the repair of injured intestine.

3. *Gastrointestinal regulating effects*

Clinical research shows that Huoxiang Zhengqi preparations can treat senile abdominal distension; the drug can regulate gastrointestinal dysfunction and has a two-way regulating effect on gastrointestinal motility. It also promotes digestion and absorption, relieving stomach distension and diarrhea. It can also enhance the intestinal propulsion function of normal mice, and has a significant excitatory effect on atropine to inhibit the small intestinal movement of mice, and has a significant inhibitory effect on neostigmine-induced small intestinal movement excitement in mice. It shows that Huoxiang Zhengqi preparations have a two-way regulating effect on the movement of the small intestine in mice.

4. *Anti-emetic effects*

Huoxiang Zhengqi preparations have anti-vomiting and anti-emetic effects, which can prolong the incubation period of vomiting and reduce the amount of vomiting in pigeons.

5. *Anti-inflammatory effects*

Huoxiang Zhengqi preparations can be used to treat type allergic diseases clinically. Animal experiments *in vitro* confirmed that Huoxiang Zhengqi water can inhibit passive allergic reaction in rats, inhibit antigen–antibody reaction, stabilize mast cell membrane, block mast cell degranulation and release mediator, reduce inflammation, and improve cell structure and function. Huoxiang Zhengqi water has the function of releasing drugs from allergic reaction medium, so it can prevent antigen–antibody reaction and prevent pathological damage caused by an inflammatory medium.

6. *Antiviral effects*

Flavonoids in Cablin Potchouli Herb can resist the growth and reproduction of viruses, and hesperidin in Tangerine Peel can prevent cold virus infection, but the antiviral activity is eliminated by hyaluronidase. The glycyrrhizin in liquorice root has the effect of inhibiting the proliferation of HIV. Glycyrrhiza Polysaccharide has obvious effects against vesicular stomatitis virus, adenovirus, herpes simplex virus type, and vaccinia virus, and can inhibit the occurrence of cytopathic diseases.

7. *Bacteriostatic effects*

Huoxiang Zhengqi water has different degrees of antibacterial effects on eight kinds of bacteria such as Sarcina lutea, Staphylococcus aureus, Shigella, and Salmonella, especially a stronger effect on Sarcina lutea and Staphylococcus aureus, and has a strong bacteriostatic effect on Shigella, *Bacillus proteus*, *Trichophyton rubrum*, *Trichophyton Mentagrophytes*, *Acrothesium floccosum*, *Trichophyton cerebriformis*, *Microsporum gypseum*, *Candida albicans*, *Cryptococcus neoformans*, *Blastomycosis dermatitidis*, and *Bacillus paratyphosus* A and B.

8. *Improving water, electrolyte, and metabolic disorders*

An animal model of sub-healthy rats with a syndrome of dampness retaining in the spleen and stomach was established. After Huoxiang Zhengqi powder was administered, it was confirmed that it can increase serum glucose, protein, and lipid content and reduce serum Na^+, K^+, and Cl^- levels to improve nutrient absorption and metabolic function. Huoxiang Zhengqi water can also increase the expression of AQP4 mRNA in the intestinal mucosa of rats with spleen deficiency and dampness stagnation syndrome, and enhance the absorption of water by the colon.

9. *Tranquilizing effects*

Huoxiang Zhengqi has an inhibitory effect on spontaneous activity in mice. The main herb (Cablin Potchouli Herb) can expel wind-cold, resolve dampness with aromatics, and regulate the stomach and spleen. It can be supplemented with Pinellia Tuber for calming and sedative effects; Perilla Leaf and Dahurian Angelica Root for the effect of invigorating the spleen for eliminating dampness; and Areca Peel for the effect of activating qi-flow and removing dampness.

The combined use of all these medicines has the effects of dispelling wind, eliminating evils, and harmonizing the stomach, so it can play the role of eliminating pathogens and strengthening vital qi, regulating the balance of the body, and promoting the automatic tranquilization of Yang qi to achieve the effect of Yin and Yang intersection, which is desirable for sleep.

III. Pharmacist's Notes

(1) It is not advisable to take tonic Chinese medicines while taking this medicine.

(2) This product contains Pinellia Tuber. It has been reported that overdose or prolonged use of Pinellia Tuber has strong irritation on local mucous membranes, causing chronic poisoning. Other possible consequences include renal compensatory enlargement with the liver and intestine as other toxic target organs. Pathological examination does not show obvious pathological morphological changes. In addition, it has gestational embryotoxicity and teratogenic effects.

Therefore, it should be taken strictly in accordance with the administration and dosage, and should not be taken in excess or for a prolonged period. If there are adverse reactions or discomfort after taking the drug, the drug should be discontinued, and those with severe symptoms should see a doctor in time.

(3) It is prohibited for those allergic to this product; use with caution for allergic individuals.

(4) Huoxiang Zhengqi water contains alcohol, and is prohibited for people with alcohol allergies.

(5) Huoxiang Zhengqi water contains alcohol. After taking the drug, it is not advisable to drive a vehicle such as a plane, car, or boat, and it is also not advised to work at a height, operate machinery or precision instruments.

(6) Huoxiang Zhengqi water contains alcohol; avoid taking other drugs that may produce disulfiram-like reactions.

(7) This product is mainly used to treat common cold caused by cold-dampness or summer-heat dampness. It is recommended for those with fatigue and gastrointestinal discomfort during the medical observation period. This product is especially suitable for those with fatigue, diarrhea, and abdominal pain. For those with fatigue and fever, it is recommended to use Jinhua Qinggan granule, Lianhua Qingwen capsule (granule), and Shufeng Jiedu granule.

(8) Avoid smoking, alcohol, and spicy, cold, greasy foods while taking this medicine, and a light diet is preferred.

(9) Patients with severe chronic diseases, such as high blood pressure, heart disease, liver disease, diabetes, and kidney disease, pregnant women, or patients undergoing other treatments should take this medicine under the guidance of a physician.

(10) Children, pregnant women, and lactating women should use this medicine with caution under the guidance of a doctor; elderly and frail people should take this medicine under the guidance of a doctor.

(11) Patients should go and see a doctor if the symptoms have not improved, or if there is obvious vomiting and diarrhea, and other serious symptoms are present after taking the medicine for three days.

(12) It is forbidden to use when the properties of this product are changed.

(13) Children must use this medicine under the supervision of an adult.

(14) Keep this product out of the reach of children.

(15) If you are using other drugs, please consult your physician or pharmacist before using this product.

Section 2: Jinhua Qinggan Granule (see Table 3)

Boxed Warning:

This product contains Ephedra Herb (*Herba Ephedrae*), Thunberg Fritillary Bulb (*Bulbus Fritillariae Thunbergii*) and other ingredients; take caution with compatibility issues and special population medication. This product is contraindicated for allergic individuals and those who are allergic to this product.

【Ingredients】 Honeysuckle Flower (*Flos Lonicerae*), Gypsum (*Gypsum Fibrosum*), honey-processed Ephedra Herb, fried Bitter Apricot Seed (*Semen Armeniacae Amarum*), Baical Skullcap Root (*Radix Scutellariae*), Weeping Forsythia Capsule (*Fructus Forsythiae*), Thunberg Fritillary Bulb, Common Anemarrhena Rhizome (*Rhizoma Anemarrhenae*), Great Burdock Achene (*Fructus Arctii*), Sweet Wormwood Herb (*Herba Artemisiae*), Peppermint (*Herba Menthae*), and Liquorice Root (*Radix Glycyrrhizae*).

【Description】 Light brown to brown particles, slightly fragrant, and slightly bitter.

【Actions】 Ventilating lung qi, clearing heat, and removing toxicity. It is used for mild simple influenza, and wind-heat invading lung syndrome according to the pattern diagnosis of traditional Chinese medicine. Symptoms include fever, headache, body aches, sore throat, cough, aversion to wind or cold, stuffy and runny nose, red tongue, thin yellow fur, and rapid pulse.

【Indications】

(1) Influenza A H1N1;
(2) Influenza and wind-heat invading lung syndrome.

【Administration and Dosage】

Take warm after mixing the granules with boiling water, 3 times a day. The course of treatment is 3 days.

【Strengths】 5 g/sachet.

【Side Effects】

Note: Based on the summary of observed clinical adverse events, this section aims to present a comprehensive profile of all possible safety events of this product, and does not include specific data about the prevalence, severity, and scope of adverse events or adverse reactions (ADEs/ADRs).

(1) Gastrointestinal system: nausea, vomiting, diarrhea, heartburn, poor appetite can be seen.
(2) Abnormal liver function, palpitations, or rash after drug withdrawal may occur occasionally.

I. Drug–Drug Interactions Among Concomitant Medications

1. *Concomitant medications*

1.1. *The "eighteen clashes" in the combined use of Chinese herbal medicine*

This product contains Thunberg Fritillary Bulb, which is contraindicated in combination with Aconitum carmichaeli Debx; the ingredient Liquorice Root is contraindicated in combination with Seaweed (*Sargassum*), Peking euphorbia root (*Radix Euphorbiae Pekinensis*), Lilac Daphne Flower Bud (*Flos Genkwa*), and Gansui Root (*Radix Kansui*).

1.2. *Combined use of Western medicines*

(1) The combination of liquorice root in this product and aspirin causes aggravation of gastrointestinal diseases. Aspirin is irritating to the gastric mucosa, and liquorice root has a glucocorticoid-like effect, which can increase gastric acid secretion, reduce gastric mucus secretion, and reduce the resistance of the gastrointestinal tract, thus inducing or aggravating stomach and duodenal ulcers.
(2) The ephedra contained in this product, in combination with western drugs containing cardiac glycosides such as digitalis and digoxin, can increase the toxicity, and is likely to cause arrhythmia and heart failure and other toxic reactions. When taken with monoamine oxidase

inhibitors such as furazolidone and glibenclamide, the release of norepinephrine and neurotransmitters will be increased, resulting in a sudden increase of blood pressure and even hypertensive crisis.

2. Recommendations

This product contains ingredients such as fritillary bulb and ephedra. Attention should be paid to the "eighteen clashes" concerning the combined use of fritillary bulb with other medicines, and the adrenaline-like effect of ephedrine. Ephedrine can excite sympathetic nerves, relax bronchial smooth muscle, contract blood vessels, and has a significant central nervous stimulant effect, so careful consideration should be given to the combined use with Western medicines to prevent repeated medications.

II. Pharmacological Action

1. Antiviral effects

Honeysuckle Flower, Baical Skullcap Root, Weeping Forsythiae Capsule, and Sweet Wormwood Herb in this product have antiviral effects.

2. Anti-inflammatory effects

This product can significantly reduce the serum CRP and IFN-γ levels in patients, suggesting the decrease in inflammation response after treatment.

3. Immunity-enhancing effects

IFN-γ and CRP are sensitive cytokines that reflect the body's immune function. Increased concentrations of both indicate severe inflammation. Research showed that the serum CRP and IFN-γ levels of patients significantly decreased, suggesting that the patients' inflammatory reaction after treatment was reduced and the immune function improved. This may be related to the antiviral effects of Honeysuckle Flower, Baical Skullcap Root, Weeping Forsythiae Capsule, and Sweet Wormwood Herb in Jinhua Qinggan granules. The serum IFN-γ level decreased, the patient's antiviral immune response decreased, the respiratory inflammatory response caused by neutrophils and monocytes decreased, and immune function increased.

III. Pharmacist's Notes

(1) It is not advisable to take tonic Chinese medicines while taking this medicine.

(2) Ephedra Herb in this product can raise blood pressure, and athletes should use it with caution.

(3) Ephedra Herb can cause cardiovascular system toxicity (acute myocardial infarction, severe hypertension, myocarditis, arrhythmia, different types of single ventricular tachycardia, etc.) and liver toxicity (acute and chronic hepatitis, jaundice, etc.); long-term use causes central nervous system toxicity such as hallucinations, cramps, stroke, headache and insomnia, and rise of blood pressure. Therefore, patients with hypertension and heart disease should use this with caution. Blood pressure must be monitored when taking medication.

(4) Those who are allergic to this product are prohibited to take this medicine.

(5) The usual dosage recommended for Jinhua Qinggan granule is its proper dosage. Increasing the dosage will not improve the therapeutic effect.

(6) Athletes and those with deficient cold in the spleen and stomach should use the product with caution.

(7) People with a history of liver disease or abnormal liver function before taking medication should use it with caution.

(8) Avoid tobacco, alcohol, and spicy, cold, greasy food.

(9) There are no research data to support the use of this product for those with body temperature $\geq 39.1°C$, white blood cell count (WBC) $> 11.0 \times 109/L$, neutrophil ratio $> 75\%$, or severe influenza. These groups should use it under the guidance of a physician.

(10) Pregnant women, lactating women, children and the elderly should use it under the guidance of a physician.

Section 3: Lianhua Qingwen Capsule (Granule) (see Table 3)

Boxed Warning:

> **This product contains Ephedra Herb (*Herba Ephedrae*), Rhubarb (*Radix et Rhizoma Rhei*), and other ingredients; be wary of compatibility problems and special population medication. This product is contraindicated for allergic individuals and those who are allergic to this product.**

【Ingredients】 Weeping Forsythiae Capsule (*Fructus Forsythiae*), Honeysuckle Flower (*Flos Lonicerae*), honey-fried Ephedra Herb, fried Bitter Apricot Seed (*Semen Armeniacae Amarum*), Gypsum (*Gypsum Fibrosum*), Indigowoad Root (*Radix Isatidis*), Male Fern Rhizome (*Rhizoma Dryopteridis*), Heartleaf Houttuynia Herb (*Herba Houttuyniae*), Cablin Potchouli Herb (*Herba Pogostemonis*), Rhubarb, Integripetal Rhodiola Herb (*Herba Rhodiolae*), menthol, Liquorice Root (*Radix Glycyrrhizae*).

【Actions】 Clearing away pestilential toxins, ventilating the lung, and clearing heat.

【Indications】 It is used to treat influenza with syndrome of heat-toxicity blocking the lung. Symptoms include fever or high fever, aversion to cold, muscle aches, nasal congestion, runny nose, cough, headache, sore and dry throat, red tongue, and yellow fur or yellow greasy fur.

Different dosage forms of Lianhua Qingwen have different quality specifications, descriptions, administration and dosage, and strengths. See Table 2 for details.

【Side Effects】

Note: Based on the summary of observed clinical adverse events, this section aims to present a comprehensive profile of all possible safety events of this product, and does not include specific data about the prevalence, severity, and scope of adverse events or adverse reactions (ADEs/ADRs).

Table 2. Comparison of Lianhua Qingwen preparations of different dosage forms.

	Lianhua Qingwen Capsule	Lianhua Qingwen Granule
Quality Specification	Pharmacopoeia of the People's Republic of China (2015 edition one)	State Food and Drug Administration standards YBZ01632006
Description	This product is a hard capsule; the content is brownish yellow to yellowish brown granules and powder, slightly fragrant, slightly bitter	This product is brownish yellow to dark brown particles, slightly fragrant and slightly bitter
Administration and Dosage	Oral, 4 capsules at a time, 3 times a day	Oral, 1 bag at a time, 3 times a day
Strengths	0.35 g/capsule	6 g/sachet

Clinical reports of major adverse reactions/adverse events of Lianhua Qingwen capsule include nausea, vomiting, gastrointestinal discomfort, abdominal distension, diarrhea, and gastrointestinal reactions. The adverse reactions of gastrointestinal system damage mainly occur 3 hours (the longest 24 hours) after administration, and mostly affect those who have taken the medicine on an empty stomach; the adverse reactions to skin and appendage damage mainly occur within 30 minutes following medication, and often occur after taking the medicine for the first time. After taking a meal or symptomatic treatment, the adverse reactions improved or disappeared, and the prognosis was favorable.

I. Drug–Drug Interactions Among Concomitant Medications

According to the clinical reports, Lianhua Qingwen is often used in combination with the following two types of drugs: combined with oseltamivir, acyclovir, ribavirin, adenosine monophosphate, interferon, and other antiviral drugs for the treatment of viral influenza, herpangina, upper respiratory syncytial virus, pediatric hand-foot-mouth disease, herpes zoster, and other diseases; combined with antibiotics such as cephalosporins, ofloxacin, macrolides, and carbapenems for the treatment of bacterial pneumonia.

It is reported in the literature that the chemical components contained in Lianhua Qingwen capsule mainly include forsythiaside A, forsythiaside I, forsythiaside H, forsythiaside E, D-amygdalin, L-amygdalin, liriodendrin, 3,4-dihydroxybenzaldehyde, quercetin, Liquiritin apioside, isoliquiritigenin, naringenin, rhein, etc., covering phenylpropanoids, anthraquinones, flavonoids, pentacyclic triterpenes, iridoids, and other traditional Chinese medicine chemical components. Attention should be paid to avoid the drug–drug interaction caused by the combination of western medicine and traditional Chinese medicine containing the abovementioned chemical components.

1. *Issues in concomitant medications*

Rhubarb in this product contains tannin, which can bind with vitamins B to affect its absorption. It can form compounds with calcium that are difficult to be absorbed, which affects the efficacy.

Ephedrine contained in honey-fried Ephedra Herb in this product when combined with western medicines containing cardiac glycosides such as digitalis and digoxin increases toxicity and is likely to lead to arrhythmia and heart failure. Taking monoamine oxidase inhibitors such as Furazolidone and Glibenclamide at the same time will increase the release of norepinephrine and neurotransmitters, resulting in a rise in blood pressure and even hypertension crisis.

2. *Recommendations*

During the combined use of this product with other drugs, the adrenaline-like effect of ephedrine should be considered. Ephedrine can excite sympathetic nerves, relax bronchial smooth muscle, contract blood vessels, and has a significant central nervous stimulant effect, so careful consideration should be given to its combination with Western medicines to prevent repeated medications.

II. Pharmacological Action

1. *Antiviral effects*

Lianhua Qingwen has inhibitory effects on the influenza virus, parainfluenza virus 1 (HVJ-1), respiratory syncy-tial virus (RSV), adenovirus 3 and 7 (ADV3 and ADV7), herpes simplex virus 1 (HSV-1) and 2, SARS virus, etc. Randomized controlled trials of Lianhua Qingwen and the antiviral drug Oseltamivir show that Lianhua Qingwen capsule has a similar antiviral effect and even performs better in symptom relief. Lianhua Qingwen can inhibit H7N9, H1N1, and other viruses, and can reduce the generation of plaque after human or avian influenza virus infection.

Lianhua Qingwen inhibits the early stage of viral infection (0–2 hours) and inhibits viral-induced NF-κB activation in a dose-dependent manner, reducing viral-induced IL-6, IL-8, TNF-α, IP10, and MCP-1 gene expression.

2. *Antibacterial effects*

Lianhua Qingwen has a certain inhibitory effect on *Staphylococcus aureus, hemolytic streptococcus A, Streptococcus haemolyticus B, Pneumococcus, and Influenza Bacillus*, and its mechanism of action is related to the inhibition of the formation of bacterial biofilms.

3. *Immune Regulatory effects*

Experimental studies have shown that Lianhua Qingwen can significantly enhance the T lymphocyte subsets $CD4^+$ and $CD4^+/CD8^+$ in mice infected with the influenza virus, and can increase the expression of IFN-γ in the lungs of mice, thereby improving the body immune status.

4. *Antipyretic and anti-inflammatory effects*

The clinical use of Lianhua Qingwen in the treatment of acute suppurative tonsillitis showed that the average body temperature, white blood cell count, and C-reactive protein return to normal significantly sooner than those in the conventional western medicine penicillin plus ribavirin group. Pharmacological experiments show that Lianhua Qingwen can remove inflammatory factors such as interleukin-6 (IL-6) and CRP, and can strengthen the role of leukocytes.

5. *Other effects*

In vitro experiments show that Lianhua Qingwen capsule can inhibit the proliferation of breast cancer MCF-7 cells and induce apoptosis.

III. Pharmacist's Notes

(1) This product is a preparation containing Ephedra Herb, which has a central nervous stimulant effect. It should not be combined with sedative and hypnotic western medicines, which will reduce each other's efficacy; it should not be taken together with antihypertensive drugs to avoid reduction of the effect of the antihypertensive. It should not be used in combination with the monoamine oxidase inhibitors pargyline, furazolidone, amphetamine, phenylethylhydrazine, etc., as combinations cause headache, dizziness, nausea, dyspnea, and other adverse reactions and even hypertension crisis and cerebral hemorrhage for severe cases. It should not be used together with aminophylline, which can increase the toxicity of aminophylline and can cause upper abdominal discomfort or adverse reactions of the central nervous system. Athletes, patients with high blood pressure, and those with heart disease should use it with caution. Drug monitoring should be strengthened for those with severe chronic diseases such as liver disease, diabetes, and kidney disease.

(2) This product contains Rhubarb, which can regulate qi-flowing for resolving stagnation and has strong medicinal properties. Use with caution during pregnancy.

(3) Use with caution in patients with hypertension or heart disease. Those with severe chronic diseases such as liver disease, diabetes, and kidney disease should take it under the guidance of a physician.

(4) Children, pregnant women, lactating women, and those who are elderly, frail, and suffering from persistent loose stools should take it under the guidance of a physician.

(5) Children should take the medicine under adult supervision.

(6) This product has a bacteriostatic effect. It should not be taken at the same time as Western medicines containing active bacteria such as lactase.

(7) This product has certain gastrointestinal adverse reactions. It is recommended to take it after meals. If rash, edema, and other adverse reactions occur after taking the drug, the drug must be discontinued in time and medical attention should be given immediately.

(8) Avoid tobacco, alcohol, and spicy, cold, greasy food.

(9) It is not advisable to take nourishing Chinese medicines at the same time as taking this medicine.

(10) Those with common cold caused by pathogenic wind-cold should be cautious when using this medicine.

(11) Patients with fever and body temperature exceeding 38.5°C should go to the hospital for treatment.

(12) Take strictly according to usage and dosage. This product should not be taken for a prolonged period.

(13) For those who are allergic to this product and those with allergies should use it with caution.

(14) After opening the moisture-proof bag, please keep it moisture-free.

Section 4: Shufeng Jiedu Capsule (see Table 3)

Boxed Warning:

> This product is contraindicated for those who are allergic to this product.

【**Ingredients**】 Giant Knotweed Rhizome (*Rhizoma Polygoni Cuspidati*), Weeping Forsythiae Capsule (*Fructus Forsythiae*), Indigowoad Root (*Radix Isatidis*), Chinese Thorowax Root (*Radix Bupleuri*), Dahurian Patrinia Herb (*Herba Patriniae*), European Verbena (*Herba Verbenae*), Reed Rhizome (*Rhizoma Phragmitis*), Liquorice Root (*Radix Glycyrrhizae*).

【**Quality Specification**】 China Food and Drug Administration (National Medical Products Administration, or NMPA) Standard: YBZ00652009.

【**Description**】 It is a hard capsule; the contents are dark brown to brown granules or powder with fragrance and bitter taste.

【**Actions**】 Dispelling wind and clearing heat, removing toxicity, and relieving sore throat.

【**Indications**】 Acute upper respiratory tract infection with wind-heat syndrome with symptoms including fever, aversion to wind, pharyngalgia and headache, stuffy nose, runny nose, and cough.

【**Administration and Dosage**】 Four capsules orally per time, three times a day.

【**Strengths**】 0.52 g per capsule.

【**Side Effects**】

Note: Based on the summary of observed clinical adverse events, this section aims to present a comprehensive profile of all possible safety events of this product, and does not include specific data about the prevalence, severity, and scope of adverse events or adverse reactions (ADEs/ADRs).

(1) Occasional nausea.
(2) There were clinical reports of adverse reactions occurring such as facial edema and skin rash after the first administration. Other adverse reactions include bellyache, diarrhea, nausea, and other gastrointestinal discomfort.

I. Drug–Drug Interactions Among Concomitant Medications

According to the clinical reports, Shufeng jiedu capsule is often used in combination with the following two types of drugs: antivirotics (such as ribavirin, ganciclovir, and oseltamivir) for the treatment of upper respiratory tract virus infection, viral keratitis, and hand-foot-mouth disease; antibiotics (such as cephalosporins, penicillin, and quinolones) for the treatment of infectious pneumonia, otitis media, and skin diseases. There have also been reports of combined use with cimetidine in the treatment of childhood mumps.

It has been reported that the Shufeng jiedu capsule contains chemical ingredients such as alkaloids, anthquinones, flavonoids, triterpenoid saponins, phenylethanosides, iridoids, phenolic acids, and coumarins. Take caution to avoid the combination with western medicines that may trigger drug–drug interaction among the chemical ingredients stated above.

II. Pharmacological Action

1. *Antiviral effects*

The in vitro experiments of Shufeng jiedu capsule showed its inhibition effect on influenza A H1N1 (FM1 strain, PR8 strain, jiangxi pruning strain, B10 strain, and B59 strain), the parainfluenza virus (sendai strain), RSV, HSV-1, HSV-2, COX-B4, and COX-B5. The in vivo experiments showed it could act against weight reduction in mice caused by RSV infection to some extent; reduce lung swelling, lung index, and mortality in mice infected by RSV, HSV-1, and CVB3; and increase survival time and the life extension rate of experimental mice.

2. *Antibacterial effect*

Shufeng jiedu capsule can effectively inhibit the growth of *staphylococcus aureus, Escherichia coli, pseudomonas aeruginosa, shigella dysentery, streptococcus pneumoniae*, and *beta streptococcus*, presenting a broad spectrum of antibacterial effect.

3. *Antipyretic effect*

Shufeng jiedu capsule can significantly inhibit the levels of inflammatory factors (PGE2) and cytokines (TNF-radiation, il-1 radiation, il-1 radiation, and il-6), and reduce the values of such thermogenic media as cAMP/cGMP, the amount of cAMP, Na^+, K^+-atpase and heat production, increasing the amount of endogenous antipyretic medium AVP, so as to play its antipyretic role.

4. *Anti-inflammatory and immunomodulatory effects*

The results of network pharmacology analysis showed that the key compounds (such as nucleoside adenosine, phenolic acids, caffeic acid, anthraquinones, emodin and rhein, cycloalkene ether terpenoids verbena glycosides and phenylethyl alcohol glycosides mullein indican, licorice flavonoid glycosides, and 7-methoxy rhamnetin) of Shufeng Jiedu capsule acted on the signal pathway related to inflammation and immunomodulation by binding to the corresponding target protein. The drug can also significantly inhibit the expression and secretion of inflammatory factors in mouse lung tissue induced by pseudomonas aeruginosa or peritoneal macrophages induced by lipopolysaccharide.

Besides, its active ingredient, verbena protein, also displayed a significant anti-inflammatory effect possibly through G protein-coupled receptor 18. In addition, the metabolic pathway of arachidonic acid (AA) may be one of the important pathways for Shufeng jiedu capsule to play an anti-inflammatory and immunomodulatory role.

5. *Analgesic effect*

The hot-plate test of mice showed that Shufeng jiedu capsule had some analgesic effects.

III. Pharmacist's Notes

(1) This product contains alkaloids, which may lead to the increase of the toxicity when used in combination with alkaline Western medicine

such as aminopyrine, antipyrine, and procaine. Meanwhile, alkaloids can precipitate with heavy metal-containing western medicines (such as mercury preparations), which may affect drug absorption.

(2) This product has an antibacterial effect and should not be taken together with western medicine containing active bacteria such as lactasine.

(3) It is inadvisable to use this drug with tonic or nourishing Chinese medicine.

(4) This product can lead to gastrointestinal reactions, such as nausea and diarrhea. It is recommended for patients to take it after meals.

(5) If there are some adverse reactions (such as rash and edema) after taking this product, stop the drug and seek medical advice in time.

Table 3. Novel coronavirus pneumonia commonly used in medical observation period.

Serial number	Name of drug	Dosage form	Specifications	Functional Indications and Indications	Usage and Dosage	Matters needing attention
1	Huoxiang Zhengqi capsule	Capsule	0.3 g × 30 grain/box	It can relieve the exterior and remove dampness, regulate qi and balance the body.	Take orally, four capsules a day, twice a day.	1. It is not suitable to take tonic Chinese medicine at the same time, such as Shengxuebao mixture. 2. It is forbidden to use this product in case of allergic constitution. Children, pregnant women and lactating women should use it with caution. The elderly and the weak should take it under the guidance of doctors. 3. During taking medicine, avoid smoking, alcohol and spicy, raw and cold, greasy food, and diet should be light. 4. Patients with severe hypertension, heart disease, liver disease, diabetes, kidney disease and other chronic diseases, pregnant women or patients undergoing other treatment should be taken under the guidance of doctors. 5. This product contains Pinellia ternate and should not be used with Aconitum containing traditional Chinese medicine. 6. Huoxiang Zhengqi water contains alcohol. It is forbidden for those who are allergic to alcohol. At the same time, we should be cautious in combination to avoid disulfiram like reaction. 7. Huoxiang Zhengqi water contains alcohol. After taking medicine, it is not allowed to drive aircraft, vehicles, boats, or engage in aerial work, mechanical work and operation of precision instruments.
2	Huoxiang Zhengqi pill	Pills	Concentrated pill: each 8 pills is equivalent to 3 g of the original drug; Water pill: 6 g/pouch; Drop pills: 2.6 g/pouch	It is used for cold caused by exogenous wind cold, dampness stagnation of internal injury or summer dampness. The symptoms include headache, dizziness, chest and diaphragmatic distension, abdominal distension and pain, vomiting and diarrhea. It is also used for gastrointestinal diseases such as functional dyspepsia, postoperative flatulence, irritable bowel syndrome, acute gastroenteritis, diabetic diarrhea, viral enteritis, gastric or duodenal ulcer, acute and chronic colitis, etc.	Concentrated pill: Oral, 8 pills a time, 3 times a day. Water pill: Oral, 6 g a time, twice a day. Drop pills: Oral, 1–2 pouches, twice a day.	
3	Huoxiang Zhengqi water	Tincture	10 ml/bottle		Oral, 5–10 ml, twice a day, shake well.	
4	Huoxiang Zhengqi oral liquid	Mixture	10 ml/bottle			

| 5 | Jinhua Qinggan granules | Granule | 5 g × 6 Pouches/box | Dispersing wind and dispersing lung, clearing away heat and detoxification. It is used for fever, aversion to cold, mild or not averse to cold, red throat, stuffy nose, runny nose, thirst, cough or phlegm caused by exogenous pathogenic factors, etc. It is suitable for all kinds of influenza, including influenza A H1N1. | Take it with boiling water, 1 bag at a time, twice a day, for 3–5 days. | 1. Avoid spicy, raw and cold, greasy food, diet should be light.
2. It should be used with caution for those who have cold, cold and sore throat, no sweat and clear nose.
3. This product contains ephedra, hypertension, heart failure, glaucoma, immune deficiency and other patients with caution.
4. It is not suitable to take tonic Chinese medicine at the same time, such as Shengxuebao mixture. |
| 6 | Lianhua Qingwen capsule | Capsule | 0.35 g × 24 grains/box | It can clear away pestilence and detoxify, and release lung heat. It is used to treat epidemic febrile fever and fever, aversion to cold, muscle soreness, nasal congestion and runny nose, cough, headache, dry throat and sore throat, red tongue, yellow or yellow greasy fur. | Oral, 4 capsules a time, 3 times a day. | 1. It is not suitable to take tonic Chinese medicine at the same time, such as Shengxuebao mixture.
2. This product contains ephedra, hypertension, heart disease patients with caution.
3. This product is bitter and cold, easy to hurt the stomach qi. It should be taken under the guidance of doctors for the elderly, weak, children, pregnant women, lactating women, patients with spleen deficiency and loose stool. |

(Continued)

Table 3.   *(Continued)*

Serial number	Name of drug	Dosage form	Specifications	Functional Indications and Indications	Usage and Dosage	Matters needing attention
7	Lianhua Qingwen granule	Granule	6 g 10 Pouches/box	It can clear away pestilence and detoxify, and release lung heat. It is used to treat epidemic febrile fever and fever, aversion to cold, muscle soreness, nasal congestion and runny nose, cough, headache, dry throat and sore throat, red tongue, yellow or yellow greasy fur.	Oral, 1 bag at a time, 3 times a day.	1. It is not suitable to take tonic Chinese medicine at the same time, such as Shengxuebao mixture. 2. This product contains ephedra, hypertension, heart disease patients with caution. 3. This product is bitter and cold, easy to hurt the stomach qi. It should be taken under the guidance of doctors for the elderly, weak, children, pregnant women, lactating women, patients with spleen deficiency and loose stool.
8	Shufeng Jiedu Capsule	Capsule	0.52 g × 48 grains/box	Dispelling wind and clearing heat, relieving sore throat and detoxication. For acute upper respiratory tract infection, it belongs to wind heat syndrome. The symptoms include fever, evil wind, sore throat, headache, nasal congestion, turbid runny nose, cough, etc.	Oral, 4 capsules a time, 3 times a day.	1. It is not suitable to take tonic Chinese medicine at the same time, such as Shengxuebao mixture. 2. This product is bitter and cold, easy to hurt the stomach qi. It should be taken under the guidance of doctors for the elderly, weak, children, pregnant women, lactating women, patients with spleen deficiency and loose stool.

Chapter 5

Guidance on Rational Application of Chinese Patent Medicine during Clinical Treatment Period

The *Diagnosis and Treatment Protocol for Novel Coronavirus Pneumonia* (Trial Version 7) issued by the National Health Commission and National Administration of Traditional Chinese Medicine recommend the use of eight Chinese Patent Medicines [Xiyanping Injection, Tanreqing Injection, Xuebijing Injection, Xingnaojing Injection, Reduning Injection, Shengmai Injection, Shenfu Injection, and Shenmai Injection] for the treatment of severe and critical cases in the clinical treatment period.

Section 1: Xiyanping Injection (see Table 1)

Boxed Warning:

> This product is contraindicated for those who are allergic to this product, women during pregnancy, and children under 1 year old.

【Ingredients】 Total sulfonates of andrographolide.

【Quality Specification】 China Food and Drug Administration (National Medical Products Administration, or NMPA) Standard: WS-10863 (ZD-0863)-2002-2011Z.

【Description】 It is a yellowish to yellow-green transparent liquid for injection.

【Actions】 Clearing heat and removing toxicity, relieving cough and dysentery.

【Indications】 Bronchitis, tonsillitis, bacillary dysentery, etc.

I. Administration and Dosage

(1) Intramuscular injection: 50 ~ 100 mg per time for adults, 2 ~ 3 times a day; for pediatric use, reduce the dose as advised by healthcare providers.
(2) Intravenous drip: Adults: Total daily dosage ranges between 250 and 500 mg per day. Dilute the dose with 100 ml ~ 250 ml 5% glucose or 0.9% sodium chloride solution. Maintain the dripping rate within the range of 30 ~ 40 drops per minute. One infusion per day; otherwise, follow the healthcare provider's advice.

Children: A total daily dosage of 5 ~ 10 mg/kg (0.2 ~ 0.4 ml/kg) or 2.3 ~ 4.5 mg/lb (0.09 ~ 0.18 ml/lb) per day with the maximum daily dosage not exceeding 250 mg.

【Strengths】 2-ml ampoule: 50-mg therapeutic agent;

5-ml ampoule: 125-mg therapeutic agent.

【Side Effects】

Note: Based on the summary of observed clinical adverse events, this section aims to present a comprehensive profile of all possible safety events of this product, and does not include specific data about the prevalence, severity, and scope of adverse events or adverse reactions (ADEs/ADRs).

According to the reports by China National ADEs/ADRs Surveillance Center, allergic events of this product top the list of all ADEs/ADRs events, followed by the respiratory, cardiovascular, and dermatological symptoms. Children under 14 years of age are the population with the most frequently reported ADEs/ADRs events, including adverse reactions such as allergy, anaphylactic shock, cyanosis, and dyspnea.

(1) Allergic events: erythema, skin rash, pruritus, dyspnea, palpitations, cyanosis, decreased blood pressure, swollen larynx, or even anaphylactic shock and pre-shock manifestations, such as cyanosis of lips, weak pulse, and cold limbs.

(2) Skin and appendages: urticaria, maculopapule, erythematous eruption, piebaldness, wheal, flushed skin, scleroma, local swelling, angioedema, etc.

(3) Systemic reactions: chills, shivering, fever, pallor, hidrosis, cold sweating, pain, fatigue, edema, etc.

(4) Digestive system: nausea, vomiting, diarrhea, abdominal pain, abdominal distension, xerostomia, stomach upset, abnormal liver biochemical parameters, urinary and fecal incontinence, paroxysmal abdominal pain, hyperactive bowel sounds, watery stools, etc.

(5) Respiratory system: chest pain, chest distress, breathlessness, tachypnea, coughing, sneezing, laryngeal itching, laryngeal stridor, nasal congestion, wheezing rales present in both lungs, laryngeal constriction, etc.

(6) Cardiovascular system: palpitations, chest distress, chest pain, tachycardia, arrhythmias, etc.

(7) Nervous system: dizziness, headache, convulsion, numbness, tremor, vertigo, tinnitus, dysphoria, drowsiness, insomnia, psychentonia, obnubilation, trismus, tetanic convulsion of limbs, etc.

(8) Vision: binocular gaze, blurred vision.

(9) Urinary system: renal failure, anuria.

(10) Local reactions: skin rashes, pain, numbness, itching, phlebitis, etc.

II. Drug–Drug Interactions Among Concomitant Medications

According to the ADR case report, Xiyanping Injection is often used in combination with the following five types of drugs: antibiotics, antivirals, nutrients, antiallergic agents, and other traditional Chinese medicine (TCM) injections. Antibiotics are the most commonly used type of concomitant medication.

1. *Issues of concomitant medications*

It has been observed that after mixing Xiyanping Injection with ambroxol injection for 3–5 min, the solution becomes cloudy and white crystals may appear. Further experiments indicate that this occurs when Xiyanping Injection is diluted with either one of 11 solvents including antibiotic (ambroxol hydrochloride, dexamethasone sodium phosphate, vitamin B6, levofloxacin, cefoperazone sodium, cefoperazone sulbactam sodium, ceftazidime, azithromycin injections) and antiviral agents (ribavirin, acyclovir, ganciclovir, etc.). The increased number of non-soluble particles has exceeded the relevant provisions of the Pharmacopoeia of the People's Republic of China.

In addition, after the combination of Xiyanping Injection and the sodium chloride solvent, the number of particles also increased.

2. *Recommendations*

The combined application of Xiyanping Injection and other drugs mainly affects the stability of the infusion, and the resulting particles may block the local vessels, leading to phlebitis, edema, and allergic reactions. Xiyanping Injection's package insert indicates that "there have been no data about the interaction between this product and other drugs". However, the precautions clearly point out that it is strictly prohibited to mix products in clinical safe use.

Xiyanping Injection, as a traditional Chinese medicine preparation with complex ingredients, should be used with caution concomitantly with other medical administration. If combination therapy is needed, the concentration of drugs and interval duration between different products should be taken into careful consideration, and it is recommended to flush the infusion tube when changing medicine. They can also be administered separately, without sharing the same venous pathway, or after a drug is infused, normal saline or 5% glucose injection can be used as the insulating infusion to prevent drug–drug interactions.

In the treatment of COVID-19, the combination of Xiyanping Injection and oral administration of traditional Chinese medicine decoction can be considered for severe cases with pattern of flaring heat in qi and ying aspects.

III. Pharmacological Action

1. *Antiviral effects*

The in vitro tests of Xiyanping injection showed the inactivation effect on adenovirus III (ADV3), influenza A virus I, influenza A virus V, influenza A virus III, respiratory syncytial virus (RSV), etc.

Mechanism: Xiyanping Injection is composed of total sulfonates of andrographolide, which is highly concentrated in the blood and penetrates virus cells well. It adheres to the binding sites for viral DNA replication and protein expressions, prevents protein from wrapping the DNA fragments, and makes the virus unable to replicate, thus inhibiting or killing the virus.

2. *Antibacterial effects*

Xiyanping injection has significant bactericidal and bacteriostatic effects on Gram-positive bacteria (enteropathogenic E.coli, *Salmonella typhi*, *Streptococcus pneumoniae*, *Haemophilus influenzae*, *Staphylococcus aureus*, *Hemolytic streptococcus*) and some gram-negative bacteria (*Proteus*, *Shigella dysenteriae*). In addition, animal experiments showed that it has a significant protective effect on mice infected with *Staphylococcus aureus* and *Streptococcus pneumoniae*.

3. *Antitussive effects*

Xiyanping Injection can inhibit the cough incubation period induced by citric acid, and has a significant inhibitory effect on the number of coughs in guinea pigs.

Mechanism: It can relax the smooth muscle of the trachea and bronchus, relieve the spasm of smooth muscle, and inhibit the secretion of serous fluid, helping to expectorate phlegm and relieve cough.

4. *Anti-inflammatory and antipyretic effects*

Mechanism: Experiments on the effects of Xiyanping Injection on the cytokine levels in bronchoalveolar lavage fluid (BALF) of rats with LPS-induced acute lung injury reveal that it plays an anti-inflammatory role by inhibiting the release of proinflammatory factors. Meanwhile, it can inhibit the synthesis of prostaglardin in the inflammatory site, protect the lysosome membrane, decrease the inflammatory exudate, and improve the capillary circulation, achieving the anti-inflammatory effect.

In addition, Xiyanping Injection has an antipyretic effect on the fever caused by endotoxin, pneumococcus, and hemolytic streptococcus. Xiyanping Injection can reduce the temperature set point to the normal level by inactivating the endogenous pyrogen, such as interleukin-1, interleukin-6, and tumor necrosis factor.

5. *Immunity-enhancing effects*

Mechanism: Xiyanping Injection can boost immunity by promoting adrenocortical function, enhancing phagocytosis of macrophages and neutrophils, and increasing the lysozyme content in serum. Besides, it can also improve the level of serum properdin, increase the T and B cell density in the spleen, and promote the formation of immunoglobulin.

IV. Pharmacist's Notes

(1) Anaphylactic shock can occur as the adverse reactions of this product, so this product should be used in settings of medical institutions with resuscitation facilities and personnel. Healthcare providers should have received anaphylactic shock rescue training. If there is any allergic reaction or other serious adverse reactions, administration of this product should be discontinued immediately and first aid treatment should be given in a timely manner.

(2) This product shall be used in strict accordance with indications described in the package insert. Off-label application is prohibited.

(3) The administration and dosage should strictly follow the instructions listed in the package insert. Use the recommended dosage. Overdose, excessively fast infusion, and long-term continuous medication are not allowed.

(4) This product is a traditional Chinese medicine injection, whose quality can be affected by improper storage. The product should be checked carefully before use, during preparation, and during administration. It is not allowed to use if some changes of drug properties (turbidity, sediment, discoloration, crystallization) or some damage of the bottle (air leak, crack) is present.

(5) Xiyanping Injection should be used with caution in combination with other drugs. If combined use is needed, the concentration and interval time between different drugs should be carefully considered, and it is recommended to flush the infusion tube when changing medicine to prevent possible drug–drug interactions.

(6) Before administration, the patient's condition, medication history, and allergy history should be inquired. This drug should be used with caution and under close surveillance for older patients, lactating women, children, patients with family allergy history, allergic constitution, abnormal liver and kidney function, and patients who use this TCM injection for the first time.

(7) This product is prohibited to use for children under 1 year of age. Children between 1 and 2 years of age should use this product with caution.

(8) Medication monitoring should be strengthened. During the course of administration, the drug reaction should be closely observed, especially for the first 30 minutes. If there is any abnormal event, administration of this product should be discontinued immediately and the patient should be treated with necessary measures.

(9) The mixture of Xiyanping Injection and 5% glucose injection or 0.9% sodium chloride injection is stable within 4h, so it is recommended to administer the mixture within 4h after preparation.

(10) Xiyanping Injection can be used in severe and critical cases of COVID-19 with heat patterns. If the fever has subsided, it should be promptly stopped to prevent possible damage to patients' yang qi.

Section 2: Tanreqing Injection (see Table 1)

Boxed Warning:

This product is contraindicated for those who are allergic to this product and alcohol, elderly patients with liver and kidney dysfunction, severe cor pulmonale with heart failure, women during pregnancy, and children under 2 years old.

【Ingredients】 Baical Skullcap Root (*Radix Scutellariae*), Bear Gall Powder (*Fel Ursi*), Cornu Caprae Hircus (*Naemorhedus goral Hardwicke*), Honeysuckle Flower (*Flos Lonicerae*), Weeping Forsythiae Capsule (*Fructus Forsythiae*); the excipient is glycol propylene.

【Quality Specification】 National Drug Standard: YBZ00912003-2007Z-2009-2012.

【Description】 It is a brown-red liquid for injection.

【Actions】 Clearing heat, resolving phlegm, and removing toxicity.

【Indications】 Wind-warm disease with lung heat with syndrome of phlegm and blood stasis obstructing lung, symptoms including fever, cough, expectoration difficulty, sore throat, thirst, red tongue, yellow fur; early stage of pneumonia, acute bronchitis, acute attack of chronic bronchitis, and upper respiratory tract infection with the abovementioned syndromes.

I. Administration and Dosage

(1) Adults: 20 ml per time under normal circumstances, 40 ml per time for severe patients. When using this product, add 5% glucose injection or 0.9% sodium chloride injection 250 ~ 500 ml. Intravenous drip once a day at a rate of no more than 60 drops per minute.

(2) Children: The dose should be converted according to 0.3 ~ 0.5 ml/kg, and the maximum dose should not exceed 20ml. When using this product, add 5% glucose injection or 0.9% sodium chloride injection 100 ~ 200 ml. Intravenous drip once a day at a rate of 30 ~ 60 drops per minute or follow the doctor's advice.

【Strengths】 10 ml: ampoule.

【Side Effects】

Note: Based on the summary of observed clinical adverse events, this section aims to present a comprehensive profile of all possible safety events of this product, and does not include specific data about the prevalence, severity, and scope of adverse events or adverse reactions (ADEs/ADRs).

According to the report, most of the ADR events mainly involve damage to the skin and appendages, and the proportion of systemic reactions, damages to the digestive system, cardiovascular system, nervous system, and other systems, was similar. From January 2014 to May 2015, using the design scheme of a cohort study combined with a case–control study and the form of drug-induced prospective hospital centralized monitoring, the safety of Tanreqing injection was evaluated for a total of 30322 emergency patients in 93 hospitals, and the overall incidence of adverse reactions was 0.27% without serious adverse reaction.

A small number of patients may have dizziness, chest tightness, nausea, vomiting, and diarrhea. Some patients had color flush, rash, or pruritus occasionally. Palpitations, shivering, and dyspnea are rare; anaphylactic shock is even rarer. Other adverse reactions: dry mouth, fever, periorbital and facial edema, discomfort of injection site, etc.

(1) Skin and appendages: rash, itchy skin, wheal, urticaria, erythema, maculopapules, blisters, facial swelling, periorbital edema.
(2) Cardiovascular system: palpitations, atrial fibrillation, arrhythmia, decreased blood pressure, chest tightness, chest pain, cyanosis, purpura, phlebitis.
(3) Nervous system: headache, dizziness, disultiplam-like reactions, anxiety and garrulousness, local or systemic numbness, tremor, dizziness, convulsions, confusion.
(4) Systemic reactions: chill, fever, aversion to cold.
(5) Digestive system: nausea, vomiting, bellyache, diarrhea, abdominal distension, constipation, upset stomach, dry mouth.
(6) Peripheral blood vessels: phlebitis, facial flushing.
(7) Respiratory system: dyspnea, laryngeal spasm, laryngeal edema, gurgling with sputum in throat, pharyngeal itch, breathlessness, tachypnea, cough, nasal congestion, runny nose.

(8)   Vision: blurred vision.
(9)   Urinary system: dysuria, anuria, or hematuria.
(10) Musculoskeletal reactions: arthralgia, myalgia.
(11) Local reactions: rash, pain, or other reactions at the injection site.
(12) Allergic events: fever, chills, sweating, cyanotic lips and limbs, coolness of extremities, flushed complexion, dysphoria, obnubilation, loss of consciousness, swollen lip, eyelid edema, pricking in eyes, blurred vision, pallor, hoarseness, and anaphylactic shock.

As for the causes of adverse reactions, it is considered that some of the ingredients of Tanreqing injection, such as the baicalin in Baical Skullcap Root, cholalic acid in Bear Gall powder, hydrolysate in Cornu Caprae Hircus, chlorogenic acid in Honeysuckle Flower, and phillyrin in Weeping Forsythiae Capsule, can cause allergic reactions. The chlorogenic acid and hydrolysate of Cornu Caprae Hircus are known to be hypersensitive, which may easily lead to many types of allergic reactions.

II. Drug–Drug Interactions Among Concomitant Medications

1. *Issues in concomitant medications*

According to clinical application and experimental studies, the main problem involved in the combination of Tanreqing Injection with other drugs is producing precipitation particles, resulting in safety risk in intravenous injection. The results of literature evaluation showed that Tanreqing Injection is often used in combination with the following five types of drugs: anti-infective drugs, respiratory drugs, digestive drugs, vitamin, and electrolyte. The experimental results showed that Tanreqing Injection reacted with almost all quinolones, the hydrochlorate, lactate and mesylate of levofloxacin, some aminoglycosides, few cephalosporins, and had almost no reaction with penicillin.

The drugs or solvents mixed with Tanreqing injection that can produce turbidity or precipitation: gentamicin, ciprofloxacin, vitamin B6, levofloxacin, gatifloxacin, pazufloxacin, pefloxacin, ornidazole, fluconazole, acyclovir, ganciclovir, tobramycin, vancomycin, cephalosporins, cefamandole, cefepime, albomycin, azithromycin, clindamycin, vitamin

K3, bromhexine, Aspirin/lysine, compound amino barbitone and reduced glutathione, calcium gluconate, 10% invert sugar, 10% fructose, mannitol, glycerin fructose sodium chloride, sugar mixed electrolyte potassium, sodium, magnesium, calcium and glucose, methoxychlor amine, and aminomethylbenzoic acid.

The drugs mixed with Tanreqing injection that can produce turbidity or precipitation, which would not dissolve after being heated: Tobramycin sulfate, gentamicin sulfate, and 10% calcium gluconate. These drugs are contraindicative in compatibility.

The drugs mixed with Tanreqing injection that can produce turbidity or precipitation that dissolve after being heated and reappear after cooling: vancomycin, albomycin, azithromycin, gatifloxacin, sodium lactate ciprofloxacin, pefloxacin mesilate, levofloxacin hydrochloride, levofloxacin mesylate, parazloxacin mesylate, cefotiam, cefepime, cefamandole, fluconazole, bromhexine hydrochloride, acyclovir injection, ganciclovir injection, lincomycin hydrochloride, reduced glutathione, aspisol, vitamin B6, vitamin K3, reclomide. These drugs are contraindicated in combination use.

2. Recommendations

The use of Tanreqing injection in combination with other drugs mainly affects the stability of the infusion and the content of active ingredients, and the sediment can block the local blood vessels, leading to phlebitis, edema, and allergic reactions. Tanreqing Injection's package insert indicates that "there have been no data about the interaction between this product and other drugs". However, the precautions clearly point out that it is strictly prohibited to mix with other products in clinical use.

In view of the problems of the combined use of Tanreqing injection with other drugs, pharmacists suggested that the drug can be used in combination with other drugs as follows:

(1) Tanreqing injection contains various complex and sensitizing ingredients. It should be used with caution concomitantly with other medical administration. If a combination is needed, the concentration of drugs and interval duration between different products should be taken into careful consideration, and it is recommended to flush the infusion tube when changing medicine. They can also be administered

separately without sharing the same vascular access, or after a drug is infused, normal saline or 5% glucose injection can be used as the insulating infusion to prevent drug-to-drug interactions.

(2) Tanreqing injection can be combined with penicillin and most cephalosporins, but not with quinolones. Avoid the use of drugs that have compatibility contraindications with Tanreqing injection as mentioned above.

(3) The stability of Tanreqing injection is related to the pH value, and it is sensitive to acidic liquid with pH < 6, which is likely to cause precipitation. Therefore, drastic change in pH should be avoided when combined with other drugs. When used in combination with antibiotics, the pH value is generally required to be between 6 and 8. If the pH value is less than 6 or more than 8, the application is not recommended, so as to avoid the changes caused by the reaction of the two ingredients, which may threaten the health or even life.

(4) In the treatment of COVID-19, the combination of Tanreqing injection and traditional Chinese medicine decoction can be considered for the severe syndrome of flaring heat in qi and ying aspects.

III. Pharmacological Action

1. *Antibacterial and antiviral effects*

The *in vitro* tests showed that Tanreqing injection could inhibit *streptococcus pneumoniae*, beta *hemolytic streptococcus, staphylococcus aureus*, and *influenzae haemophilus*. This product can reduce the mortality rate of mice infected by staphylococcus aureus and the influenza virus, and reduce the viral hemagglutination titer in lung homogenate, showing an inhibitory effect on the virus.

Mechanism: This product can induce the production of interferon-α in the lung tissue of mice infected with the influenza virus, and can cause a significant promotion in the proliferation of T cells and B cells and the phagocytosis of peritoneal macrophages.

Moreover, it can release the inhibited state of IL-4 secretion by Th2 cells in the lung homogenate of virus-infected mice, and promote the secretion of Th1 by IFN-jerk. In addition, this product can reduce TNF-α content in alveolar lavage fluid in the rat model of inflammation infected by endotoxin and the mice infected with the influenza virus.

2. *Anti-inflammatory and antipyretic effects*

Tanreqing injection can inhibit the formation of inflammatory granuloma in rats and ear swelling of mice caused by xylene, and can reduce the body temperature of rabbits infected by endotoxin and rats infected by yeast.

Mechanism: Tanreqing injection has a corresponding effect on macrophages and neutrophils in the body, so as to effectively enhance the anti-inflammatory effect. Meanwhile, it can increase the content of serum lysozyme in the blood, thus reducing the duration of lung rums. Furthermore, this product can inhibit the inflammatory exudation and pulmonary interstitial edema, inhibit or reduce the infiltration of inflammatory cells, prevent the injury of acute alveolar cell inflammation, and relieve the hypoxic state. It can also reduce the expression level of the endotoxin inflammatory cytokines, inhibit the production of central febrile mediators PGE2 and cAMP, inhibit the expression of inflammatory cytokines (such as TNF-α, IL-1, IL-6, IL-8, and IL-17α) on protein and mRNA levels, promote the differentiation of Th2 cells, and improve the level of anti-inflammatory factor IL-4, so as to achieve the anti-inflammatory effect.

3. *Antitussive effects*

Tanreqing injection can increase the phenol red excretion of the mice's trachea and prolong the incubation period of cough induced by ammonia and sulfur dioxide. The in vivo experiments showed that Tanreqing injection could significantly inhibit the excessive production of MUC5AC, which is the main component of airway mucus stimulated by LPS.

4. *Spasmolysis*

Tanreqing injection shows the inhibition of convulsion in mice induced by strychnine nitrate and valedrazole.

5. *Immunity-enhancing effects*

Mechanism: Tanreqing injection can significantly increase CD4, CD8, and NK cells, and promote the production of serum antibodies, thus enhancing the immune function.

6. *Apoptosis-promoting effects*

Tanreqing injection can inhibit the proliferation of leukemic cells in vitro.

Mechanism: Tanreqing injection reduces the proportion of S phase, downregulates the expression of apoptosis-related gene bcl-2, and upregulates the expression of caspase-3.

IV. Pharmacist's Notes

(1) Anaphylactic shock can occur as a very rare adverse reaction of this product, so this product should be used in settings of medical institutions with resuscitation facilities and personnel. During the process of administration, patients' reactions should be closely observed, especially in the first 5–30 minutes. If there is any allergic reaction or other serious adverse reactions after administration, administration of this product should be discontinued immediately and first aid treatment should be given in a timely manner. The residual liquid and all the equipment used for infusion should be properly kept after the patient's use. Blood samples should be collected and refrigerated to facilitate the possible subsequent tracing of the cause of adverse reactions.

(2) This product shall be used in strict accordance with indications described in the package insert. Off-label application is prohibited. This product is used for the treatment of wind-warm disease with lung heat that is categorized as the syndrome of heat-phlegm obstructing lung and common cold with wind-heat syndrome, and it is not used for the treatment of the syndrome of cold-phlegm obstructing the lung and common cold with wind-cold syndrome. In the clinical use, we should pay attention to the syndrome differentiation of cold and heat and apply it rationally.

(3) The administration and dosage should strictly follow the instructions listed in the package insert. Use the recommended dosage, preparation requirements, and speed of infusion. Excessively fast infusion and long-term continuous medication are not allowed.

(4) The temperature of the dilution solvent should be appropriate to ensure that the liquid is at room temperature during infusion, generally at 20 ~ 30. The dilution ratio of liquid medicine should be no less than 1:10 (medicine:solvent), so it is recommended to administer the mixture within 4h after preparation. Carefully check the drug and the

dispensed liquid before administration. If the drug solution is found to be turbid, or sediment, discoloration, crystallization, or other changes are found in drug properties, bottle cap leakage as well as slight fracture of bottle, the injection shall not be used.

(5) Tanreqing Injection should be used with caution in combination with other drugs. If combined use is needed, the infusion tube should be flushed with 5% glucose injection or 0.9% sodium chloride injection (above 50 ml) or replaced with a new infusion set when changing medicine. In addition, the concentration and interval time between different drugs should be carefully considered to prevent possible drug-to-drug interactions.

(6) In the process of infusion, if bubbles are present when the liquid passes through the filter, the dripping rate should be slowed down. Strictly control the infusion speed: 30 ~ 40 drops per minute for children and 30 ~ 60 drops per minute for adults. A very fast dripping rate or leakage can cause dizziness, chest distress, or local pain.

(7) Before administration, the patient's condition, medication history, and allergy history should be inquired. This drug should be used with caution and under close surveillance for older patients, lactating women, children, patients with family allergy history, allergic constitution, and patients who use this TCM injection for the first time.

Section 3: Xuebijing Injection (see Table 1)

Boxed Warning:

> **This product is contraindicated for those who are allergic to this product, women during pregnancy, and children under or during 14 years old.**

【Ingredients】 Safflower (*Flos Carthami*), Red Peony Root (*Radix Paeoniae Rubra*), Szechuan Lovage Rhizome (*Rhizoma Chuanxiong*), Danshen Root (*Radix Salviae Miltiorrhizae*), Chinese Angelica (*Radix Angelicae Sinensis*); the excipients are glucose and polysorbate 80 (for injection).

【Quality Specification】 China Food and Drug Administration (National Medical Products Administration, or NMPA) Standard: YBZ01242004-2010Z-2012.

【Description】 It is a brown-yellow transparent liquid for injection.

【Actions】 Expelling blood stasis and detoxification.

【Indications】 Fever-related diseases with symptoms including fever, shortness of breath, heart palpitations, irritability, and other syndromes of blood stasis and toxins, systemic inflammatory response syndrome induced by infection, and be used in combination with other drugs to treat organ dysfunction in multiple organ dysfunction syndrome.

I. Administration and Dosage

(1) Systemic inflammatory response syndrome: Intravenous infusion of 50 ml plus 100 ml of 0.9% sodium chloride injection, finished within 30–40 minutes, twice a day; three times per day for severe cases.

(2) Multiple organ malfunction syndrome: Intravenous infusion of 100 ml plus 100 ml of 0.9% sodium chloride injection, finished within 30–40 minutes, twice a day; three or four times a day for severe cases.

【Strengths】 10 ml: ampoule.

【Side Effects】

Note: Based on the summary of observed clinical adverse events, this section aims to present a comprehensive profile of all possible safety events of this product, and does not include specific data about the prevalence, severity, and scope of adverse events or adverse reactions (ADEs/ADRs).

(1) Allergic events: erythema, skin rash, pruritus, dyspnea, palpitations, cyanosis, increased or decreased blood pressure, swollen larynx, anaphylactic shock, etc.

(2) Systemic reactions: shivering, fever, pallor, fatigue, hidrosis, cold sweating, convulsion.

(3) Skin and appendages: skin anaphylactic response, skin rashes, pruritus, flushed skin.

(4) Cardiovascular system: palpitations, cyanosis, increased or decreased blood pressure, arrhythmias.

(5) Nervous system: dizziness, headache.

(6) Respiratory system: dyspnea, chest distress, breathlessness, tachypnea, coughing, swollen larynx.

(7) Digestive system: nausea, vomiting, abdominal pain, diarrhea, fecal occult blood, abnormal liver biochemical parameters.

(8) Urinary system: frequent micturition, urgent urination, dysuria, hematuria.

(9) Injection site: redness and swelling, pain.

(10) Others: edema of face, conjunctival congestion, abnormal lacrimation, phlebitis, lumbago, backache, local numbness.

II. Drug–Drug Interactions Among Concomitant Medications

Xuebijing Injection is mainly used to treat systemic inflammatory response syndrome and multiple organ dysfunction syndrome, and is often applied in combination with hormone drugs and antibacterial drugs.

1. *Issues in mixed administration*

1.1 *The "eighteen clashes" in the combined use of Chinese herbal medicine*

This product contains Danshen Root, Peony Root; according to the compatibility taboo of "eighteen clashes", Falsehellebore Root and

Rhizome (*Radix et Rhizoma Veratri*) are incompatible with all types of Red Paeony Root and White Paeony Root (*Radix Paeoniae Alba*). So, it should not be used in combination with drugs containing Falsehellebore Root and Rhizome.

1.2 Combined use of Western medicines

When Xuebijing Injection is combined with hydrocortisone, ceftriaxone sodium, levofloxacin, or penicillin sodium, the index components show a tendency to degrade after compatibility. After being directly combined with ceftriaxone sodium, put it at room temperature. The color of the solution gradually deepens (from light yellow to reddish brown) with time, and it is close to reddish brown 8 hours later; when it is used in combination with other injections, the mixture often becomes cloudy.

2. Recommendations

Xuebijing Injection, as a traditional Chinese medicine preparation with complex ingredients, should be administered on the basis of TCM theory, and be used strictly in accordance with the functional indications and recommended dosages in the package insert. It is strictly forbidden to mix with other drugs directly. If combination therapy is needed, flush the infusion tube with 50-ml normal saline when changing medicine, and keep a certain interval time. In addition, pay attention to the principle of "eighteen clashes" compatibility taboo.

III. Pharmacological Action

1. Improving blood coagulation

This product can reduce the mortality of mice caused by endotoxin and improve the coagulation function of disseminated intravascular coagulation (DIC) model rats. Mechanism: Increase the content of fibrin and platelets in model rats, shorten the time of prothrombin and thrombin, increase the aggregation rate of platelets, and reduce the content of plasma thromboxane B2 (TXB2).

2. *Anti-endotoxin effects*

Treat the toxic damage to the rat liver due to endotoxin, and increase the activity of superoxide dismutase (SOD). Mechanism: Xuebijing Injection can antagonize the increase of serum TNF-α, IL-6, and IL-8 levels caused by *endotoxin* attack in mice.

3. *Phagocytosis-improving effects*

The phagocytosis index α value and clearance index K value of the mouse are activated and increased, and the phagocytic function of the reticuloen-dothelial system (RES) is enhanced.

4. *Anti-inflammatory effects*

It has a strong effect of antagonizing the uncontrolled release of inflammatory mediators and has an antagonistic effect on the increase of serum tumor necrosis factor (TNF-α) level in mice.

5. *Immune-regulating effects*

It can increase humoral immune function and increase the level of anti-sheep erythrocyte antibody in the serum of sensitized mice. Mechanism: By regulating 550 targets such as HRAS, GSK3B, BTK, and AK, acting on 10 pathways such as B cell receptor signal transduction pathway, vascular endothelial growth factor signal pathway, natural killer cell-mediated cytotoxicity, and Toll-like receptor signal transduction, it thus plays its role in anti-inflammatory and immune regulation.

6. *Protect and repair damaged organs*

Xuebijing Injection can protect the lungs, kidneys, and other organs.

IV. Pharmacist's Notes

(1) Anaphylactic shock can occur as one of the adverse reactions of this product, so this product should be used in settings of medical institutions with resuscitation facilities and personnel. Healthcare

providers should have received anaphylactic shock rescue training. If there is any allergic reaction or other serious adverse reactions after administration, administration of this product should be discontinued immediately and first aid treatment should be given in a timely manner.

(2) This product should be used on the basis of controlling the primary disease when treating systemic inflammatory response syndrome induced by infection and multiple organ dysfunction syndrome.

(3) This product must be used immediately after diluting according to the instructions.

(4) The product should be checked carefully before use, during preparation, and during administration. It is not allowed to use if some changes of drug properties (turbidity, crystallization, discoloration) or some damage of the bottle (crack) is present.

(5) The product should be used with caution in combination with other drugs. If combined use is needed, flush the infusion tube with 50-ml 0.9% sodium chloride solution when changing medicine, and keep a certain interval time.

(6) Before administration, the patient's medication history, allergy history, and family allergy history should be inquired. It is prohibited to use for people with allergic physique or those who are allergic to this product or the Safflower, Red Peony Root, Szechuan Lovage Rhizome, Chinese Angelica, and Danshen Root, and adjuvants listed in the ingredients.

(7) When using this product, it should not be combined with other Chinese medicine injections. If it is really necessary, monitoring should be strengthened.

(8) For elderly patients and patients who are using traditional Chinese medicine injections for the first time, medication monitoring should be strengthened, and the dosage and drip rate must be adjusted according to the clinical condition and physical condition.

(9) It is prohibited to use this medicine for women during pregnancy and children under or during 14 years of age.

(10) During the medication process, observe the medication response closely, especially the initial 30 minutes of intravenous infusion. Once an abnormal situation occurs, stop the medicine immediately and treat it symptomatically.

(11) 0.9% sodium chloride is the preferred solvent and the drip should be finished in 4 hours.

Section 4: Xingnaojing Injection (see Table 1)

Boxed Warning:

> This product is contraindicated for those who are allergic to this product, women during pregnancy, and children under or during 3 years old.

【Ingredients】 Musk (*Moschus*), Turmeric Root-tuber (*Radix Curcumae*), Borneol (*Borneolum*), Cape Jasmine Fruit (*Fructus Gardeniae*); the excipients are polysorbate 80 and sodium chloride.

【Quality Specification】 China Food and Drug Administration (National Medical Products Administration, or NMPA) Standard: WS3-B-3353-98-2003.

【Description】 It is a colorless and clear liquid.

【Actions】 Clearing heat and removing toxicity, cooling blood and activating blood circulation, inducing resuscitation, and restoring consciousness.

【Indications】 Apoplexy, hemiplegia and mouth skew, external injury and headache, coma, heart alcoholism, headache and vomiting, coma with convulsion caused by qi, and blood adverse flow and blood stasis in the brain vessels; including cerebral embolism, acute cerebral hemorrhage, head trauma, acute alcoholism with the syndromes mentioned above.

I. Administration and Dosage

(1) Intramuscular injection: 2 ~ 4 ml per time, 1 ~ 2 times per day.
(2) Intravenous drip: 10 ~ 20 ml per time, dilute it with 5% ~ 10% glucose injection or 0.9% sodium chloride injection to 250 ~ 500 ml, instill once a day; otherwise, follow the healthcare provider's advice.

【Strengths】 10 ml/5 ml/2 ml: ampoule.

【Side Effects】

Note: Based on the summary of observed clinical adverse events, this section aims to present a comprehensive profile of all possible safety events of this product, and does not include specific data about the prevalence, severity, and scope of adverse events or adverse reactions (ADEs/ADRs). The fastest adverse reactions occurred within 1 minute after the start of medication, the slowest occurred after 14 days of continuous medication, and the most common occurred within 30 minutes.

(1) Allergic events: erythema, skin rash, pruritus, dyspnea, palpitations, cyanosis, decreased blood pressure, anaphylactic shock, etc.
(2) Systemic reactions: chills, shivering, fever, fatigue, pain, pallor, hidrosis, etc.
(3) Respiratory system: chest distress, coughing, tachypnea, cyanosis, etc.
(4) Cardiovascular system: palpitations, tachycardia, chest distress, increased or decreased blood pressure, etc.
(5) Nervous system: dizziness, headache, convulsion, delirium, convulsion, coma, unconsciousness, mental disorder, limbs numbness, dysphoria, etc.
(6) Skin and appendages: windy skin rash, urticaria, piebaldness, exfoliative dermatitis, etc.
(7) Digestive system: nausea, vomiting, abdominal pain, diarrhea, etc.
(8) Injection site: pain, redness and swelling, numbness, skin rashes, phlebitis, etc.

II. Drug–Drug Interactions Among Concomitant Medications

1. *Issues in concomitant medications*

When continuous intravenous infusion of Xingnaojing Injection and omeprazole (losec) was administered, the drug solution in the infusion tube appeared light red. When Xingnaojing Injection is combined with 5% glucose injection, there tend to be many adverse reactions. When dissolved in other injections for infusion, the insoluble particles should be carefully checked.

2. *Recommendations*

The incidence of adverse reactions is high when using 5% glucose injection as solvent. It is recommended to choose 0.9% sodium chloride solution as the solvent. This product should be used alone; mixing or matching with other drugs is forbidden. If combination therapy is needed, problems of interval duration and possible drug–drug interactions should be given careful consideration.

III. Pharmacological Action

1. *Regulating central nervous system*

A small dose of Xingnaojing Injection can excite the central nervous system, while a large dose inhibits it, showing a two-way regulation. Low dose of Xingnao Jing Injection can significantly increase the number of free movements in mice, antagonize the sleep effect of pentobarbital sodium-induced mice, increase the convulsive mortality in mice caused by the central stimulant drug strychnine, and antagonize the respiratory depression of morphine. Large doses can reduce the number of free movements of mice, antagonize the seizures caused by strychnine, and reduce the incidence of electrical convulsions in mice.

Mechanism: Muskone in Xingnaojing Injection can inhibit vascular permeability and fight hypoxia.

2. *Brain protection*

Mechanism: Xingnaojing Injection can inhibit the expression of inflammatory factors and vascular endothelin, inhibit the inflammatory response, and regulate vascular endothelin, augustin (SOD), diastolic factors, etc., to protect the cerebral cortex ultrastructure. In addition, by reducing the expression of Bax, it can also inhibit the expression of pathological apoptosis genes and proteins to protect brain tissue.

3. *Reducing brain edema*

Mechanism: Xingnaojing Injection contains Musk and Borneol, the combination of which has a prominent effect in preventing cerebral ischemia, and can improve the permeability of the blood–brain barrier and protect the blood–brain barrier.

4. *Improving brain microcirculation*

Xingnaojing Injection can effectively reduce the patient's whole blood specific viscosity, plasma specific viscosity, wet mass, dry mass, thrombus length, erythrocyte electrophoresis time, etc., thereby effectively improving the patient's microcirculation and enhancing the therapeutic effect.

5. *Antiepileptic effects*

Xingnaojing Injection has the functions of cooling blood, clearing heat, and removing toxicity, and can play a role in awakening and sedating and as an antispasmodic for epilepsy patients, effectively reducing the number of epilepsy attacks in patients and improving the total treatment efficiency.

6. *Anti-angina effects*

Xingnaojing Injection combined with intravenous injection of glucose injection can treat angina pectoris. Borneol in Xingnaojing Injection can improve myocardial hypoxia tolerance, and Cape Jasmine Fruit can effectively decrease blood pressure. The combination of Turmeric Root-tuber, Musk, and Borneol has the effect of resuscitating and dredging collateral, activating qi and activating blood circulation, analgesia, improving blood viscosity, promoting myocardial blood supply, and oxygen balance.

IV. Pharmacist's Notes

(1) Anaphylactic shock can occur in the adverse reactions of this product, so this product should be used in settings of medical institutions with resuscitation facilities and personnel. Healthcare providers should have received anaphylactic shock rescue training. If there is any allergic reaction or other serious adverse reactions after administration, administration of this product should be discontinued immediately and first aid treatment should be given in a timely manner.

(2) This product shall be used in strict accordance with indications described in the package insert. Off-label use is prohibited.

(3) The administration and dosage should strictly follow the instructions listed in the package insert. Use the recommended dosage. Overdose, excessively fast infusion, and long-term continuous medication are not allowed.

(4) This product is a traditional Chinese medicine injection, whose quality can be affected by improper storage. The product should be checked carefully before use, during preparation, and during administration. It is not allowed to use if some changes of drug properties (turbidity, sediment, discoloration, crystallization) or some damage of the bottle (air leak, crack) is present.

(5) This product is an aromatic drug and should be used immediately after opening to prevent volatilization.

(6) Before administration, the patient's condition, medication history, and allergy history should be inquired. Caution should be taken for patients with allergies, athletes, patients with abnormal liver and kidney functions, the elderly, lactating women, and patients who are using traditional Chinese medicine injections for the first time. If it is really necessary, follow the healthcare provider's advice and strengthen monitoring.

(7) At present, there are no systematic research data on children using this product. Not recommended for children.

(8) Strengthen medication monitoring. During the medication, the medication response should be closely observed, especially in the first 30 minutes; if there is any abnormal event, administration of this product should be discontinued immediately and the patient should be treated with necessary measures.

(9) The monitoring data show that there are reports of abnormal liver biochemical indicators related to the use of this product. It is recommended to strengthen monitoring of relevant indicators during clinical use.

(10) Those who are allergic to this product or Musk, Cape Jasmine Fruit, Turmeric Root-tuber, Borneol, and the other ingredients listed and those with a history of serious adverse reactions are prohibited to use this medicine.

(11) This product contains aromatic drugs, which are forbidden for pregnant women.

Section 5: Reduning Injection (see Table 1)

Boxed Warning:

This product is contraindicated for those who are allergic to this product, women during pregnancy and lactation.

【Ingredients】 Sweet Wormwood Herb (*Herba Artemisiae*), Honey-suckle Flower (*Flos Lonicerae*), Cape Jasmine Fruit (*Fructus Gardeniae*); the excipient is polysorbate 80.

【Quality Specification】 China Food and Drug Administration (National Medical Products Administration, or NMPA) Standard: YBZ082-02005-2015Z.

【Description】 It is a yellowish brown to reddish brown transparent liquid.

【Actions】 Clearing heat, dispelling wind, removing toxicity.

【Indications】 Common cold and cough caused by exogenous wind-heat, symptoms including high fever, slight aversion to wind and cold, headache and pantalgia, coughing, yellow phlegm; upper respiratory tract infection, acute bronchitis.

I. Administration and Dosage

(1) Adults: 20 ml per time, dilute it in 250-ml 5% glucose or 0.9% sodium chloride injection; intravenous drip at the rate of 30 ~ 60 drops per minute, one infusion per day. The course of treatment for patients with upper respiratory tract infection is 3 days. For patients with acute tracheobronchitis, it is 5 days; otherwise, follow the healthcare provider's advice.

(2) Children & adolescents: for children 3–5 years of age, not exceeding 10 ml per time, dilute it in 50-ml ~ 100-ml 5% glucose or 0.9% sodium chloride solution; intravenous drip at the rate within the range of 30 ~ 40 drops per minute. One infusion per day.

For children 6 to 10 years of age, 10 mL per time, dilute the dose in 100-ml ~ 200-ml 5% glucose or 0.9% sodium chloride solution; intravenous drip at the dripping rate within the range of 30 ~ 60 drops per minute. One infusion per day.

For children 11–13 years of age, 15 ml per time, dilute the dose with 200-ml ~ 250-ml 5% glucose or 0.9% sodium chloride solution; intravenous drip at the dripping rate within the range of 30 ~ 60 drops per minute. One infusion per day.

For adolescents 14–17 years of age, 20 mL one time, dilute the dose in 250-ml 5% glucose or 0.9% sodium chloride solution; intravenous drip at the dripping rate within the range of 30 ~ 60 drops per minute. One infusion per day.

Otherwise follow the healthcare provider's advice.

【Strengths】 10 ml: ampoule.

【Side Effects】

Note: Based on the summary of observed clinical adverse events, this section aims to present a comprehensive profile of all possible safety events of this product, and does not include specific data about the prevalence, severity, and scope of adverse events or adverse reactions (ADEs/ADRs).

(1) Skin and appendages: wheal rash, flush, urticaria, maculopapule, vesicle, pruritus, redness and swelling, stabbing pain, etc.
(2) Digestive system: nausea, vomiting, abdominal pain, diarrhea, xerostomia, etc.
(3) Circulatory system: palpitations, cyanotic limbs, pale skin, etc.
(4) Nervous system: dysphoria, numbness, dizziness, headache, unconsciousness, convulsion, syncope, drowsiness, shaking hand, tinnitus, etc.
(5) Respiratory system: tachypnea, asthma, throat discomfort, chest distress, coughing, chest pain, cyanosis of lips, dyspnea, etc.
(6) Urinary system: incontinence of urine, hematuria.
(7) Systemic reactions: pallor, shivering, profuse sweating, fever, anaphylactic shock and pre-shock manifestations.
(8) Musculoskeletal and connective tissues: right rib pain, muscle tremor.
(9) Ocular area: blurred vision, blepharoedema.

(10) Local reactions: phlebitis, vesicle, pain, redness and swelling, pruritus.

(11) Others: swollen head and face, hoarseness, leucopenia.

II. Mixed Administration

Reduning Injection combined with penicillins, cephalosporins, macrolides, lincomycin, quinolones, and other antibacterial drugs can shorten the duration of fever and improve the symptoms of inflammation; combined with interferons and nucleoside antiviral drugs for the treatment of angina, herpes, and pediatric hand-foot-mouth disease, it is significantly effective and safe.

1. *Issues in concomitant medications*

Reduning Injection should not be placed in the same container with cephalosporins, quinolones, macrolides, hormones, and other antibiotics; otherwise sediment, turbidity, crystallization, etc., would occur; there may be turbidity or flocculation in Qingkailing Injection when combined with ambroxol hydrochloride, cimetidine hydrochloride, or naproxen sodium injection. Reduning Injection and its active ingredients (organic acids, iridoids, and flavonoids) have different degrees of inhibition or induction on different CYP enzymes.

2. *Recommendations*

If combined use is needed, use 0.9% sodium chloride injection (more than 50 ml) or 5% glucose injection to flush the infusion tube or replace the infusion tube before replacing the drug, and at least 10 minutes apart; use separately when used in combination with other injections with separate preparation. In addition, Reduning Injection can inhibit or induce different CYP enzymes, so it is necessary to adjust the dosage when combining Reduning Injection with drugs metabolized by related enzymes.

III. Pharmacological Action

1. *Antipyretic effects*

This product has an antipyretic effect on rat fever caused by 2,4-dinitrophenol or on Escherichia coli and rabbit fever caused by triple vaccine.

2. *Antiviral effects*

It can prolong the average survival time of influenza virus-infected mice, and it can have a certain effect on reducing the lung index of influenza virus-infected mice.

3. *Antibacterial effects*

Honeysuckle has the effect of resisting pathogenic microorganisms and has inhibitory effects on various pathogenic bacteria. It has a certain effect on reducing the mortality of Staphylococcus aureus-infected mice and Klebsiella pneumoniae-infected mice.

4. *Anti-inflammatory effects*

It can inhibit the swelling of mouse ears caused by xylene.

5. *Analgesic effects*

It can inhibit the writhing pain response of mice caused by acetic acid.

6. *Immunity-enhancing effects*

Artemisia annua extract in Reduning Injection has an immunomodulatory effect.

(1) It can improve the serum carbon particle clearance index of mice, increase the level of serum hemolysin, and enhance the delayed hypersensitivity of mice induced by sheep red blood cells.

IV. Pharmacist's Notes

(1) Anaphylactic shock can occur as one of the adverse reactions of this product, so this product should be used in settings of medical institutions with resuscitation facilities and personnel. Healthcare providers should have received anaphylactic shock rescue training. If there is any allergic reaction or other serious adverse reactions after administration, administration of this product should be discontinued immediately and first aid treatment should be given in a timely manner.

(2) This product shall be used in strict accordance with indications described in the package insert. Off-label use is prohibited.

(3) Before administration, the patient's medication history and allergy history should be inquired. This drug should be used with caution and under close surveillance for people with allergic physique, family allergy history, elderly patients, children, abnormal liver and kidney function, and patients who use this TCM injection for the first time. Patients with previous hemolysis (slightly increased blood bilirubin or positive urine bileogen) should use with caution.

(4) Mixed administration is strictly prohibited. This product should be used alone, and it is strictly forbidden to mix with other drugs in the same container.

(5) Use with caution in combination therapy. There may arise turbidity or sediment when combined with penicillins, aminoglycosides, and macrolides. If it is indeed necessary to use in combination, flush the infusion set with 5% glucose injection or 0.9% sodium chloride solution (more than 50 ml), or use a new infusion set, and keep a certain interval time, to prevent possible drug–drug interactions.

(6) The administration and dosage should strictly follow the instructions listed in the package insert. Use the recommended dosage, preparation requirements, drip rate, and course of treatment as instructed in the drug package insert. The dose, drip rate, and course of treatment should be within normal ranges; avoid prolonged and continuous use. The dilution of medicines should be prepared in strict accordance with the usage and dosage in the instructions. The amount of diluent must be more than 4 times (including 4 times) the liquid; do not change the type of diluent.

(7) Use immediately after preparation; it should not be stored for a long time.

(8) Strengthen medication monitoring. A very fast drip rate of this product may cause dizziness, chest distress, and local skin rashes. During the administration, do not exceed the prescribed drip rate, and observe the medication response closely, especially in the first 30 minutes. If there is any abnormal event, administration of this product should be discontinued immediately and the patient should be treated with necessary measures.

(9) Improper storage of this product may affect the quality. It should be carefully checked before use. It is not allowed to use if some changes of drug properties (turbidity, sediment, discoloration, air

leak) or some damage of the bottle (crack) is present. When it is diluted by 5% glucose injection or 0.9% sodium chloride solution, it should not be used if it appears cloudy.

(10) Clinical trials have shown that blood TBIL and D-BIL increased after administration. It may be related to medicines. Please test blood T-BIL and D-BIL regularly after taking medicine.

(11) It is forbidden to use for those who are allergic to the Sweet Wormwood Herb, Honeysuckle Flower, Cape Jasmine Fruit, and the ingredients listed in this product or those with a history of serious adverse reactions.

(12) This product is contraindicated for women during pregnancy and lactation.

(13) The solvent should use 0.9% sodium chloride injection or 5% glucose injection, and the infusion should be completed within 2 hours.

Section 6: Shengmai Injection (see Table 1)

Boxed Warning:

This product is contraindicated for those who are allergic to this product, women during pregnancy, and newborns and infants.

【Ingredients】 Red ginseng (*Radix Ginseng Rubra*), Dwarf Lilyturf Tuber (*Radix Ophiopogonis*), Chinese Magnoliavine Fruit (*Fructus Schisandrae*); the excipient is polysorbate 80.

【Quality Specification】 China Food and Drug Administration (National Medical Products Administration, or NMPA) Standard: WS3-B-2865-98-2011 and Pharmacopoeia of the People's Republic of China [2012] 240.

【Description】 It is a yellowish or yellowish brown transparent liquid for injection.

【Actions】 Benefiting qi and nourishing yin, restoring pulses, and rectifying collapses.

【Indications】 Palpitations, shortness of breath, coldness of limbs, sweating, and faint pulse caused by qi and yin deficiency and pulse asthenia; seen in myocardial infarction, cardiogenic shock, septic shock, etc.

I. Administration and Dosage

(1) Intramuscular injection: 2 ml ~ 4 ml per time, 1 ~ 2 times a day.
(2) Intravenous drip: Dilute the dose with 20-ml ~ 60-ml 5% glucose injection. 250 ml ~ 500 ml at a time; otherwise, follow the healthcare provider's advice.

【Strengths】 10 ml: ampoule.

【Side Effects】

Note: Based on the summary of observed clinical adverse reactions/adverse events, this section aims to present a comprehensive profile of all possible safety events of this product, and does not include specific data about the prevalence, severity, and scope of adverse events or adverse reactions (ADEs/ADRs).

From January 1st, 2004 to September 30th, 2011, 508 cases of serious adverse reactions/adverse events after Shenmai injection were reported to the case report database of the national drug adverse reaction monitoring center. The top three observed adverse reactions/adverse events were systemic damage, respiratory system, and cardiovascular system.

(1) Allergic events: flush, skin rash, pruritus, dyspnea, palpitation, cyanosis, decreased blood pressure, swollen larynx, anaphylactic shock, etc.
(2) Systemic damage: chills, fever, shivering, aversion to cold, cold sweating, fatigue, pain, pallor, etc.
(3) Skin and appendages: skin rash, pruritus, regional skin reaction, etc. Cases of exfoliating dermatitis have been reported.
(4) Digestive system: nausea, vomiting, abdominal distension, abdominal pain, diarrhea, stomach upset, xerostomia, numbness of mouth and tongue, etc.
(5) Cardiovascular system: palpitation, chest distress, chest pain, cyanosis, elevated or lowered blood pressure, arrhythmia, cardiac region discomfort, etc.
(6) Nervous system: dizziness, headache, numbness, convulsion, tremor, fullness in head, obnubilation, insomnia, mental disorder, etc.
(7) Respiratory system: dyspnea, tachypnea, coughing, asthma, laryngeal edema, throat discomfort, etc.
(8) Injection site: phlebitis, local pain, local numbness, etc.
(9) Others: low back severe pain, myalgia, bulbar conjunctiva edema, visual acuity abnormal, voiding dysfunction, periorbital edema, etc.

II. Drug–Drug Interactions Among Concomitant Medications

1. *Issues in concomitant medications*

1.1. *The "eighteen clashes" and "nineteen incompatibilities" in the combined use of Chinese herbal medicine*

This product contains red ginseng; according to the "eighteen clashes" incompatibility of drugs in prescription, Chinese medicine veratrol contraindicates any types of panax; according to the "nineteen incompatibilities" in prescription, ginseng is incompatible with trogopterus dung. Therefore, the drug should not be used in combination with drugs containing Falsehellebore Root and Rhizome (*Radix et Rhizoma Veratri*) or Trogopterus Dung (*Faeces Togopterori*).

1.2. *Combined use of Western medicines*

This product is commonly used concomitantly with 14 drugs in clinic. Although there is no significant change in appearance and clarity after combination with vitamin C injection, the pH value will change (increased by 0.2); therefore, clinical use should avoid concomitant use with Vitamin C.

2. *Recommendations*

Caution should be taken when combining medications. If combined medications are required, the concentration and time of medication and the interval between different medications should be carefully considered. It is recommended to flush the infusion tube when changing medication. After a drug is delivered, physiological saline or 5% glucose injection can be used as a spacer to prevent drug–drug interactions. They can also be infused separately without sharing the same venous pathway. At the same time, avoid combining drugs that are incompatible with Shengmai Injection.

III. Pharmacological Action

1. *Immunity-enhancing effects*

It can significantly increase the number of T cells and enhance the function of T cells. It can also enhance the phagocytic function of macrophages, improve cellular immune function, and stimulate the secretion of human corticosterone.

2. *Protecting the heart muscle*

It can increase myocardial contractility, dilate coronary artery, reduce myocardial oxygen consumption, improve myocardial metabolism, improve myocardial resistance to ischemia and hypoxia, and improve cardiac dysfunction. The mechanism is mainly to increase the levels of superoxide dismutase (SOD) and nitric oxide (NO) in the serum, while reducing the level of malondialdehyde (DAM), effectively resisting oxidation, and scavenging oxygen free radical, thereby protecting the heart muscle.

3. *Treating various shocks*

Shengmai Injection can effectively improve the blood circulation of patients by enhancing heart function, and has good therapeutic effect on cardiogenic shock, hypovolemic shock, and septic shock.

4. *Protecting liver cells*

Shengmai Injection can enhance liver detoxification function, promote liver protein and glycogen biosynthesis, regulate the body's redox system, and reduce free radical damage to liver cells.

5. *Treating pulmonary heart disease*

Shengmai Injection can improve the function of the reticuloendothelial system, thereby reducing the activity of smooth muscle cells, enhancing myocardial contractility and tissue hypoxia tolerance, and it has good therapeutic effect for patients with pulmonary heart disease.

IV. Pharmacist's Notes

(1) This product is not suitable for those with chest pain and heartache caused by cold-induced coagulation and blood stasis. It is prohibited to use for those who have lingering pathogenic heat caused by an excess pattern or summer-heat or those who cough with existing exterior pattern. It is prohibited to use for neonates, infants, and children; it should be used with caution for pregnant women, patients with a history of drug allergies or an allergic physique. Clinical monitoring should be strengthened when using this medicine for the elderly and physically frail people and patients with severe cardiopulmonary diseases.

(2)   When used in combination with other injections, the drug concentration and time, and the interval between different drugs should be considered. It is recommended to flush the infusion tube when changing drugs to prevent drug–drug interactions. When stored in natural lighting conditions for 5 hours or less, the clarity and color of Shengmai Injection in 0.9% sodium chloride injection and 5% glucose injection have no obvious changes, and there is no turbidity or precipitation. It is recommended for clinical use within 5 hours after preparation. Before infusion with Shengmai Injection, insoluble particles should be checked and qualified before use. Otherwise, the particles generated may block the local area, which may lead to phlebitis, edema, and allergic reactions.

(3)   It is recommended to use for critical cases of COVID-19 with a syndrome of internal block and external collapse. Symptoms include shortness of breath, sudden drop in body heat, restlessness, zygomatic red, sweating, red tongue, and little fur. Shengmai Injection can also be used for critical cases and convalescent cases with the syndrome of both deficiency of qi and yin. It can nourish the yin and strengthen the qi, supplementing qi and rescuing collapse. Deficiency of qi and yin manifests as loss of appetite, pallor, dry mouth and throat, dizziness, fatigue, astringent eyes, dry stools, red tongue with little coating, and a thread and rapid pulse. Shengmai Injection has one more ingredient — Chinese magnoliavine fruit — than Shenmai Injection with three medicines perfectly combined, which boosts the effect of clearing, nourishing, and astringing, respectively. It has the analogical functions of metal and water engendering each other, and sweet and sour flavors augmenting each other. The power of nourishing qi and nourishing yin is stronger than that of Shenmai Injection. Clinical use should be strictly in accordance with the indications of this product.

(4)   In addition to use according to the instructions in the usage and dosage, if the patient has underlying diseases such as diabetes, use 0.9% sodium chloride injection instead for dilution.

(5)   In clinical application, the drip rate should not be too fast. It is advisable to maintain 20–40 drops/min for children, the elderly, and physically frail people, and 40–60 drops/min for adults to prevent adverse reactions.

(6)   This product should not be used simultaneously with the traditional Chinese medicine Falsehellebore Root and Rhizome or Trogopterus Dung.

(7)   During the administration, if the patient continues to have angina, it is advisable to take nitrate drugs or follow the doctor's advice.

(8)   This product contains saponins. It is normal to produce foam when shaking, and it does not affect the efficacy.

(9)   This product is a traditional Chinese medicine preparation; improper storage may affect product quality. Sediment inspection should be conducted before use. If any abnormality such as turbidity, precipitation, discoloration, air leak, or slight rupture of the bottle is found, it should not be used. This product should also be light checked after dilution and before infusion. Do not use it if turbidity and precipitation arise. After preparation, please use within 4 hours.

(10) This product should not be mixed with other drugs in the same container. Before and after infusion of this product, the appropriate amount of diluent should be used to rinse the infusion pipeline to avoid the possible mixing of the two drugs in the pipeline before and after the infusion which might cause adverse reactions.

(11) During the initial 30 minutes of intravenous infusion, close monitoring should be performed. If adverse reactions are present, the drug should be discontinued in time and immediate treatment should follow.

(12) This product has a blood pressure elevating response, and patients with hypertension should pay attention to changes in blood pressure when using it.

(13) Anaphylactic shock can occur as one of the adverse reactions of this product, so this product should be used in settings of medical institutions with resuscitation facilities and personnel. Healthcare providers should have received anaphylactic shock rescue training. If there is any allergic reaction or other serious adverse reactions after administration, administration of this product should be discontinued immediately and first aid treatment should be given in a timely manner.

Section 7: Shenfu Injection (see Table 1)

Boxed Warning:

> **This product contains Prepared Common Monkshood Daughter Root (Radix Aconiti Lateralis Preparata) and should be used strictly in accordance with medical advice. Newborns and infants are prohibited to use this product.**

【Ingredients】 Red Ginseng (*Radix Ginseng Rubra*), Prepared Common Monkshood Daughter Root; the excipient is polysorbate 80.

【Quality Specification】 China Food and Drug Administration (National Medical Products Administration, or NMPA) Standard: WS3-B-3427-98-2013.

【Description】 It is a yellowish or yellowish brown transparent liquid for injection.

【Actions】 Restoring yang and rescuing patient from collapse, replenishing qi, and rectifying collapse.

【Indications】 Collapses (infectious, hemorrhagic, dehydration shock, etc.) due to sudden qi depletion, and it can also be used for convulsions, palpitation, cough and gasping, stomach pain, diarrhea, arthralgia caused by yang deficiency or qi deficiency, etc.

I. Administration and Dosage

(1) Intramuscular injection: 2 ml ~ 4 ml per time, 1 ~ 2 times a day.
(2) Intravenous drip: 20 ml ~ 100 ml a time, dilute in 250-ml ~ 500-ml 5% ~ 10% glucose injection.
(3) Intravenous bolus: Dilute the dose in 20-ml 5% ~ 10% glucose injection. 5 ml ~ 20 ml per time. Otherwise, follow the healthcare provider's advice.

【Strengths】 10 ml: ampoule.

【Side Effects】

Note: Based on the summary of observed clinical adverse reactions/ adverse events, this section aims to present a comprehensive profile of all possible safety events of this product, and does not include specific data about the prevalence, severity, and scope of adverse events or adverse reactions (ADEs/ADRs).

The Guangdong Provincial Adverse Drug Reaction Testing Center conducted a large sample, multi-center, non-intervention, post-marketing safety centralized test of Shenfu Injection, collected a total of 30106 case questionnaires from 28 hospitals nationwide, and the incidence of adverse reactions was 0.76%, which is a "rare" adverse reaction. The status is "normal", and there is no "serious" adverse reaction/adverse event.

(1) Allergic events: pruritus, skin rash, allergic dermatitis, pallor, palpita-tions, dyspnea, swollen larynx, palpitations, cyanosis, lowered blood pressure, etc. In severe cases, anaphylactic shock may occur.
(2) Systemic damage: chills, fever, fatigue, hidrosis, cold sweating, waist pain, etc.
(3) Nervous system: dizziness, headache, insomnia, tremor, convulsion, numbness of lips and limbs, etc.
(4) Cardiovascular system: erythema, palpitations, chest distress, tachy-cardia, arrhythmias, blood pressure fluctuations, etc.
(5) Digestive system: nausea, vomiting, abdominal distension, abdominal pain, diarrhea, xerostomia, stomach upset, liver dysfunction, etc.
(6) Respiratory system: cyanotic lips, coughing, asthma, coughing, panting, tachypnea, etc.
(7) Urinary system: urine retention, edema, etc.
(8) Others: nose bleeding, redness and pain at the injection site, phlebitis, visual abnormality, etc.

II. Drug–Drug Interactions Among Concomitant Medications

1. *Issues in concomitant medications*

(1) The "eighteen clashes" and "nineteen incompatibilities" in the combined use of Chinese herbal medicine.

This product contains Red Ginseng, Prepared Common Monkshood Daughter Root; according to the "eighteen clashes" incompatibility of drugs in prescription, Prepared Common Monkshood Daughter Root, Pinellia Tuber (*Rhizoma Pinelliae*), Snakegourd Fruit (*Fructus Trichosanthis*)[whole Snakegourd Fruit, Snakegourd eel (Trichosanthis Pericarpium), Snakegourd Seed (*Semen Trichosanthis*), Mongolian Snakegourd Root (*Radix Trichosanthis*)]; Fritillary Bulb (*Fritillaria Bulbus*)[Unibract Fritillary Bulb (*Bulbus Fritillariae Unibracteatae*), Thunberg Fritillary Bulb (*BulbusFritillariae Thunbergii*)], Japanese Ampelopsis Root (*Radix Ampelopsis*), Common Bletilla Pseudodulb (Pseudobulbus *Bletillae*), and False-hellebore Root and Rhizome (*Radix et Rhizoma Veratri*) contraindicated with all panaxes. Therefore, the drug should not be used in combination with the herbs mentioned above.

(2) Problems in combined use with Western medicine: This product should not be directly mixed with coenzyme A, vitamin K3, aminophylline, doxorubicin hydrochloride, salvia miltiorrhiza injection, omeprazole sodium for injection, or brain protein hydrolysate for injection.

2. *Recommendations*

Caution should be taken when combining medications. If combination medications are necessitated, the concentration, time of medication, and the interval between different medications should be carefully considered. It is recommended to flush the infusion tube when changing medication. After a drug is administered, physiological saline or 5% glucose injection should be used as a spacer to prevent drug–drug interactions. They can also be infused separately without sharing the same venous pathway. At the same time, avoid combining drugs that are incompatible with Shenfu Injection.

III. Pharmacological Action

1. *Anti-heart failure effects*

Reduce the concentration of inflammatory marker plasma C-reactive protein (CRP) and interleukin-6 (IL-6) levels during the development of heart failure, and improve the patient's hemorheology (Red blood cell aggregation index, platelet adhesion rate, atrial systolic blood flow rate) and heart index.

2. *Anti-myocardial ischemia-reperfusion injury* (*MI/R*)

It can increase the levels of adenosine diphosphate, adenosine triphosphate, and adenosine phosphate in the myocardial tissue of MI/R model rats, reduce the content of myocardial malondialdehyde (MDA), increase SOD activity, scavenge oxygen free radicals, and inhibit the production of lipid excess Oxides, which play a role in resisting MI/R damage by improving the mitochondrial ultrastructure.

3. *Anti-arrhythmia effects*

It can obviously improve the Na^+-K^+-ATP enzyme activity of myocardial tissues in rabbits with chronic arrhythmia, delay the appearance time of atrioventricular block, and shorten the recovery time.

4. *Anti-shock effects*

It is widely used in infectious, cardiogenic, hemorrhagic, toxic, and other shocks. It can improve the hemodynamics of cardiogenic shock in rats, reduce the content of TNF-α and IL-1β in plasma, and downregulate the mRNA expression of TNF-α and IL-1β genes, thereby reducing myocardial ischemic injury. It can reduce plasma NO and iNOS levels of cardiogenic shock in dogs, inhibit myocardial iNOS mRNA overexpression, increase myocardial blood flow, and improve hemodynamics in shock dogs.

5. *Improving myocardial energy metabolism*

It can effectively increase the content of ATP and ADP in hypertrophic cardiomyocytes, reduce the content of AMP, and enhance the energy metabolism of hypertrophic cardiomyocytes; it can also increase the content of ATP, ADP, and AMP in ischemia-reperfusion myocardial tissue and improve the energy of ischemic myocardial tissue supply.

6. *Improving microcirculation and protect vascular endothelial cells*

It can cause the diameter of the arterioles in normal animals to expand and the number of capillary crossing network points to increase, thus speeding up the blood flow. At the same time, it also has an effect on peripheral microcirculation disorders caused by epinephrine or endotoxin. It can increase the mean arterial pressure (MAP), left ventricular diastolic pressure (LVDP), left ventricular maximum systolic rate (+ Dp/dt), left ventricular end diastolic pressure (LVEDP), and left ventricular maximum diastolic rate (− Dp/dt) to improve cardiac hemodynamics in a dose-dependent manner.

IV. Pharmacist's Notes

(1) Shenfu Injection should be diluted with 5% glucose injection and 0.9% sodium chloride injection within the prescribed concentration of usage and dosage, and the stability is good within 8 hours. It is recommended to use it within 8 hours after preparation.

(2) It is recommended to use for critical cases of COVID-19 with a syndrome of internal block and external collapse while the body is in a state of exhaustion of healthy qi. The clinical manifestations are dyspnea, wheezing, or mechanical ventilation required, dizziness, dysphoria, sweating, cold limbs, dark purple tongue, thick and greasy or dry fur, and large pulses without roots. Shock can be treated with 250 ml of 0.9% sodium chloride injection plus 100 ml of Shenfu Injection.

(3) It is forbidden to use for those who have a history of allergies or serious adverse reactions to this product, and for newborns and infants.

(4) The clinical application should strictly follow the TCM theory of treatment based on syndrome differentiation. This product is mainly suitable for the syndromes of Qi deficiency and Yang deficiency. The clinical manifestations are lethargy, low voice, spontaneous sweating, intolerance of cold, pale tongue or fat or tender, and a weak pulse. This medicine should not be used for the pattern of excess heat or Yin deficiency. This product can benefit Qi and restore Yang, and can also be used for heart failure, coronary heart disease, perioperative period, and tumors, all of which fall into the category of Yang deficiency and Qi deficiency.

(5) Anaphylactic shock can occur as one of the adverse reactions of this product, so this product should be used in settings of medical institutions with resuscitation facilities and personnel. During administration, close monitoring should be performed, especially in the first

30 minutes. Once allergic reactions or other serious adverse reactions occur, the medication must be discontinued immediately, and the airway should be kept open. Oxygen inhalation and the use of adrenaline, glucocorticoids, and other treatment measures should be given in a timely manner.

(6) The usage, dosage, and course of treatment should strictly follow the instruction in the package insert. In clinical application, the dripping rate should not be too fast. When using Chinese medicine injections for the first time, the drip rate should be maintained at 20 ~ 40 drops/min for children, elderly people, and people with a weak physique, and 40 ~ 60 drops/min for adults to prevent adverse reactions. Generally, continuous use should not exceed 20 days.

(7) If diabetic patients use this product, dilute it with 0.9% sodium chloride injection. It is not recommended to use solvents other than those instructed for dilution.

(8) This product is a traditional Chinese medicine preparation. Improper storage, such as high temperature, freezing, and collision, may affect the quality of the medicine. This product and the drip solution should be carefully checked before and after preparation and use. If the drug solution is found to be turbid, precipitated, discolored, crystalline, and other changed properties, or the bottle has leaks, cracks, etc., it should not be used. After preparation, it should be used within 4 hours.

(9) This product contains saponins. It is normal to produce foam when shaking, and it does not affect the efficacy.

Section 8: Shenmai Injection (see Table 1)

Boxed Warning:

> This product is contraindicated for those who are allergic to this product or have a history of serious adverse reactions, newborns, and infants. Pregnant women should use with caution.

【Ingredients】 Red Ginseng (*Radix Ginseng Rubra*), Dwarf Lilyturf Tuber (*Radix Ophiopogonis*); the excipients are polysorbate 80 and sodium chloride.

【Quality Specification】 China Food and Drug Administration (National Medical Products Administration, or NMPA) Standard: WS3-B-3428-98-2010.

【Description】 It is a yellowish to light brown transparent liquid for injection.

【Actions】 Invigorating qi for rescuing collapse, nourishing yin for promoting production of fluid. It is used to treat shock, coronary heart disease, viral myocarditis, chronic pulmonary heart disease, and neutropenia due to deficiency of both qi and yin. It can improve the immune function of tumor patients. When combined with chemotherapy drugs, it has a certain synergistic effect and can reduce the side effects caused by chemotherapy drugs.

【Indications】 Coronary heart disease, angina pectoris, myocardial infarction, viral myocarditis, shock, chronic pulmonary heart disease, neutropenia.

I. Administration and Dosage

(1) Intramuscular injection: 2 ~ 4 ml per time, 1 time a day.
(2) Intravenous drip: 20 ~ 100 ml at a time. Dilute with 250 ~ 500-ml 5% glucose injection or direct infusion without dilution; otherwise, follow the healthcare provider's advice.

【Strengths】   100 ml: ampoule.

【Side Effects】

Note: Based on the summary of observed clinical adverse reactions/ adverse events, this section aims to present a comprehensive profile of all possible safety events of this product, and does not include specific data about the prevalence, severity, and scope of adverse events or adverse reactions (ADEs/ADRs).

According to reports in the literature, the adverse reactions of Shenmai Injection are mainly allergic reactions and infusion reactions. Symptoms include rash, facial flushing, palpitations, chest tightness, cyanosis, and other allergic reactions and infusion reactions such as fever and chills, which may cause anaphylactic shock in severe cases.

(1) Skin and appendages: skin rash, pruritus, maculopapule, urticaria, dermatitis, etc.
(2) Systemic damage: fever, chills, hidrosis, cold sweating, erythema, fatigue, anaphylactic shock, etc.
(3) Respiratory system: dyspnea, tachypnea, coughing, sneezing, breathlessness, air-way obstruction, upper respiratory tract infection, etc.
(4) Nervous system: dizziness, headache, obnubilation, dysphoria, psychentonia, etc.
(5) Digestive system: nausea, vomiting, diarrhea, abdominal pain, constipation, xerostomia, dry mouth, flatulence, hemorrhage of upper digestive tract, hepatic failure, jaundice, etc.
(6) Cardiovascular system: palpitation, chest distress, elevated blood pressure, arrhythmia, tachycardia, angina pectoris, heart failure, etc.
(7) Musculoskeletal system: musculoskeletal pain, etc.
(8) Others: phlebitis, drug-induced fever, leukocyte elevation, irritable urination, etc.

II. Mixed Administration

1. *Issues in mixed administration*

1.1. *The "eighteen clashes" and "nineteen incompatibilities" in the combined use of Chinese herbal medicine*

This product contains Red Ginseng; according to the "eighteen clashes" incompatibility of drugs in prescription, Falsehellebore Root and Rhizome

(*Radix et Rhizoma Veratri*) contraindicate any types of panax; according to the "nineteen incompatibilities" in prescription, Ginseng is incompatible with Trogopterus Dung (*Faeces Trogopterori*). Therefore, the drug should not be used in combination with drugs containing Falsehellebore Root and Rhizome or Trogopterus Dung.

1.2. *Combined use of Western medicines*

After combination with vitamin drugs, adenosine triphosphate, and coenzyme A, the pH value changes to a certain extent, and it is recommended to avoid such combinations in clinical applications. After the infusion of the solution of 100 ml of normal saline with 40 mg of pantoprazole sodium followed by a solution of 500 ml of 5% glucose injection and 80 ml of Shenmai Injection, white turbidity immediately appeared in the drip pot, which indicates that Shenmai Injection should not be used in combination with pantoprazole sodium for infusion. In addition, Shenmai Injection cannot be used simultaneously with high-sensitivity drugs such as glycerol fructose Injection and penicillins.

2. *Recommendations*

Caution should be taken when combining medications. If combination medications are necessitated, the concentration and time of medication and the interval between different medications should be carefully considered. It is recommended to flush the infusion tube when changing medication. After a drug is delivered, physiological saline or 5% glucose injection should be used as a spacer to prevent drug–drug interactions. They can also be infused separately without sharing the same venous pathway. At the same time, avoid combining drugs that are incompatible with Shenmai Injection.

III. Pharmacological Action

1. *Anti-shock effects*

It can excite the adrenal cortex system, enhance the clearance effect of the reticuloendothelial system on various pathological substances during shock, improve the blood supply of vital organs such as the heart, liver, and brain, and improve the microcirculation and anticoagulant effect.

2. Indicated for coronary heart disease, angina pectoris, myocardial infarction, viral myocarditis, pulmonary heart disease, heart failure, etc.

It can boost heart pressure, improve coronary blood flow, increase the body's ability to withstand hypoxia, reduce myocardial oxygen consumption, protect and repair myocardial cells, and has a certain anti-arrhythmic effect.

3. Indicated for various cancer patients, having obvious synergistic and detoxifying effects when combined with chemotherapy and radiotherapy

It can improve the general health of cancer patients, protect the hematopoietic function of bone marrow, and improve the immune function of the cells of tumor patients (increasing NK, LAK activity, TH/TS value, etc.), improving the rate of tumor disappearance and shrinkage.

IV. Pharmacist's Notes

(1) After the combination of Shenmai Injection with medicines such as 0.9% Sodium Chloride Injection, 5% Glucose Injection, Xylitol Injection, Dextran 40 Injection, and Glycerin Fructose Injection, there are no substantial changes in the appearance, pH value, absorbance, microparticles, etc. Therefore, Shenmai Injection can be used concomitantly with the abovementioned medicines.

(2) This product is mainly used for critical cases of COVID-19 patients with the syndrome of internal block and external collapse. The body is in a state of deficiency and almost exhaustion of vital qi. Due to an undernourishment of the heart caused by heart Qi and Yin deficiency, the patients generally suffer from chest tightness, tingling in the precordial area, palpitations, shortness of breath, dysphoria, sleep deprivation, lethargy, white complexion, red tongue, little fur, and a thread and rapid pulse; this product can also be used for coronary heart disease, angina pectoris with the abovementioned symptoms. Two infusions a day using 0.9% sodium chloride injection 250-ml plus Shenmai Injection 100 ml can act as immunosuppression. Clinical use should be strictly in accordance with the function of this product based on syndrome differentiation.

(3) Pregnant women, patients with a history of drug allergies or allergies should use with caution. Elderly people, people with a weak physique, and patients with severe cardiopulmonary diseases should use under strengthened clinical monitoring.

(4) In addition to following the instructions in the usage and dosage, it should be diluted with 0.9% sodium chloride injection when the patients have underlying disease like diabetes.

(5) In clinical application, the drip rate should not be too fast. The drip rate should be maintained at 20–40 drops per minute for children, elderly people, and people with a weak physique, and 40–60 drops per minute for adults to prevent adverse reactions. Intravenous infusion should be administered slowly while avoiding overdose, very fast infusion, and long-term continuous administration. The drip rate should be under strict control by referring to the following two tips:

(a) If diluted with a solvent, it is recommended that the dripping rate be controlled below 40 drops/min when using the drug for the first time;

(b) For direct injection of Shenmai Injection with two specifications of 50 ml per bottle and 100 ml per bottle, it is recommended to control the drip rate at 15–20 drops/per minute.

(6) During administration, if angina continues, it is advisable to take nitrate drugs or follow the doctor's advice.

(7) This product contains saponins. It is normal to produce foam when shaking, and it does not affect the efficacy.

(8) This product is a traditional Chinese medicine preparation; improper storage may affect product quality. Light inspection must be carried out before use. If abnormal conditions such as turbidity, sediment, discoloration, or air leakage or slight rupture of the bottle are found, it should not be used; after dilution of this product and before infusion, light inspection should also be carried out. This product should not be used when there is sediment. Please use within 4 hours after preparation.

(9) This product should not be mixed with other drugs in the same container. Before and after infusion of this product, the appropriate amount of diluent should be used to rinse the infusion pipeline to avoid the mixing of the two drugs in the pipeline or adverse reactions.

(10) During the initial 30 minutes of intravenous infusion, monitoring should be strengthened, and if adverse reactions are found, the drug should be discontinued in time and treatment should follow immediately.

(11) When used in emergency and critical care, the daily dosage should not be less than 200 ml; too small a dose may affect the efficacy.

(12) Anaphylactic shock can occur in the adverse reactions of this product, so this product should be used in settings like medical institutions with resuscitation facilities and personnel. Healthcare providers should have received anaphylactic shock rescue training. If there is any allergic reaction or other serious adverse reactions after administration, administration of this product should be discontinued immediately and first aid treatment should be given in a timely manner.

Table 1. Novel coronavirus pneumonia medicines commonly used in clinical treatment.

Serial number	Name of drug	Specifications	Functional indications	Usage and dosage	Matters needing attention
1.	Xiyanping injection	In each bottle: 2 ml::50 mg; 5 ml:125 mg	Clearing heat and removing toxicity, relieving cough and dysentery. For bronchitis, tonsillitis, bacillary dysentery, etc.	1. Intramuscular injection: 50–100 mg for adults, 2–3 times a day, children should reduce the dose or follow the doctor's advice. 2. Intravenous drip: 250–500 mg for adults a day, diluted with 100–250 ml of 5% glucose injection or 0.9% sodium chloride injection, and then intravenous drip is conducted. The drip rate is controlled at 30–40 drops per minute, once a day, or as directed by a doctor; children are given 5–10 mg/kg (0.2–0.4 ml/kg) a day, and the maximum dose is not more than 250 mg.	1. It is forbidden for children under 1 year of age, people allergic to this product, pregnant women, and 1–2-year-old children. 2. For patients with abnormal liver and kidney function, the elderly, lactating women, children, and patients who use traditional Chinese medicine injection for the first time, it should be used with caution. 3. The drug should be used in strict accordance with the functional indications specified in the drug instructions, and off-labal use is prohibited. Strictly control the usage and dosage. It is strictly forbidden to mix, and the medicine should be used carefully.

2.	Tanreqing injection	In each bottle 10 ml	Clearing heat, dissipating phlegm, detoxication. It is used for the syndrome of phlegm heat obstructing lung in wind warm lung heat disease. The symptoms include fever, cough, expectoration discomfort, sore throat, thirst, red tongue, and yellowish fur, acute pneumonia, early bronchitis: acute attack of chronic bronchitis, and upper respiratory tract infection manifesting the above syndromes.	1. In general, 20 ml for adults and 40 ml for severe patients. Add 250–500 ml of 5% glucose injection or 0.9% sodium chloride injection, intravenous drip, and control the dropping speed not more than 60 drops per minute, once a day. 2. For children, it should be used according to the weight of 0.3–0.5 ml/kg, and the maximum single dose should not exceed 20 ml. Add 100–200-ml 5% glucose injection or 0.9% sodium chloride injection, intravenous drip, 30–60 drops per minute, once a day, or as directed by a doctor.	1. It is forbidden to use this product for people with alcohol allergy or allergic constitution; it is forbidden for the elderly with liver and kidney dysfunction; it is forbidden for severe pulmonary heart disease with heart failure; it is forbidden for pregnant women and infants under 24 months of age. 2. The elderly, lactating women, and patients who use traditional Chinese medicine injection for the first time should use it carefully. 3. The drug should be used in strict accordance with the functional indications specified in the drug instructions, and off-labal use is prohibited. Strictly control the usage and dosage, strictly prohibit the mixture and compatibility, and carefully combine the drugs.

(Continued)

Table 1. *(Continued)*

Serial number	Name of drug	Specifications	Functional indications	Usage and dosage	Matters needing attention
3.	Xuebijing injection	In each bottle 10 ml	Detoxication and dissipate blood stasis. It can be used for warm and heat diseases, such as fever, shortness of breath, palpitation, irritability, etc. It is suitable for systemic inflammatory response syndrome induced by infection, and can also be used in the treatment of multiple organ dysfunction syndrome.	1. Systemic inflammatory response syndrome: intravenous drip of 50 ml plus 100 ml of 0.9% sodium chloride injection within 30–40 minutes, twice a day; in severe cases, three times a day. 2. Multiple organ dysfunction syndrome: 100 ml plus 100 ml of 0.9% sodium chloride injection, intravenous drip, within 30–40 minutes, twice a day; in severe cases, 3–4 times a day.	1. It is forbidden for those who are allergic to this product; it is forbidden for pregnant women and children under 14 years of age. 2. It is not suitable to be combined with traditional Chinese medicine containing Veratrum and Western medicine that reacts with this drug. 3. The drug should be used in strict accordance with the functional indications specified in the drug instructions, and off-labal use is prohibited. Strictly control the usage and dosage, strictly prohibit the mixture and compatibility, and carefully combine the drugs.

| 4. | Xingnaojing Injection | In each bottle 10 ml/ 5 ml/2 ml | Clearing heat and removing toxicity, cooling blood and activating blood circulation, resuscitation and restoring consciousness. It is used for apoplectic coma, hemiplegic mouth deviation, traumatic headache, mental coma, alcohol poisoning, headache and vomiting, coma and convulsion caused by Qi and blood disorder and cerebral pulse stasis obstruction, cerebral embolism, acute cerebral hemorrhage, craniocerebral trauma, and acute alcoholism. | 1. Intramuscular injection: 2–4 ml once, 1–2 times a day. 2. Intravenous drip: 10–20 ml once a time, diluted with 250–500 ml of 5–10% glucose injection or 0.9% sodium chloride injection, once a day, or as directed by a doctor. | 1. It is forbidden for those who are allergic to this product; it is forbidden for pregnant women and children under 3 years of age. 2. For athletes, patients with liver and kidney dysfunction, the elderly, lactating women, and patients who use traditional Chinese medicine injection for the first time, it should be used with caution. 3. This product is an aromatic drug. It should be used immediately after opening to prevent volatilization. |

(*Continued*)

Table 1. (*Continued*)

Serial number	Name of drug	Specifications	Functional indications	Usage and dosage	Matters needing attention
5.	Reduning injection	In each bottle 10 ml	Clearing heat dispelling wind detoxication. It is used for cold and cough caused by exogenous wind heat, such as high fever, slight evil wind cold, headache, body pain, cough, and phlegm yellow; upper respiratory tract infection and acute bronchitis can see the above syndromes.	1. Adult dose: 20 ml, diluted with 250 ml of 5% glucose injection or 0.9% sodium chloride injection, intravenous drip at the rate of 30–60 drops per minute, once a day; the course of treatment for patients with upper respiratory tract infection is 3 days, and the course of treatment for patients with acute tracheobronchial inflammation is 5 days; or, follow the doctor's advice. 2. Children's dose: 3–5 years of age, the maximum dose is not more than 10 ml, 5% glucose injection or 0.9% sodium chloride injection diluted 50–100 ml, intravenous drip rate is 30–40 drops per minute,	1. It is forbidden for those allergic to this product; it is forbidden for pregnant women and lactating women; it should be used with caution if hemolysis (slight increase of blood bilirubin or positive urine bilirubin) occurred in the past. 2. The drug should be used in strict accordance with the functional indications specified in the drug instructions, and off-label use is prohibited. Strictly control the usage and dosage, strictly prohibit the mixture and compatibility, and carefully combine the drugs.

once a day; 6–10 years of age, 10 ml once a time, diluted with 5% glucose injection or 0.9% sodium chloride injection 100–200 ml, intravenous drip speed is 30–60 drops per minute. For 11–13 years of age, 15 ml of 5% glucose injection or 0.9% sodium chloride injection diluted with 200–250 ml injected intravenously at the rate of 30–60 drops per minute, once a day; for 14–17 years of age, 20 ml once a time, diluted with 250 ml of 5% glucose injection or 0.9% sodium chloride injection, the infusion rate at 30–60 drops per minute, 1 day. Or, follow the doctor's advice.

(Continued)

Table 1. *(Continued)*

Serial number	Name of drug	Specifications	Functional indications	Usage and dosage	Matters needing attention
6.	Shengmai Injection	In each bottle 10 ml	Benefiting qi and nourishing yin, rescuing patient from collapse. It is used for palpitation, shortness of breath, chills of limbs, perspiration, weak pulse, etc., caused by deficiency of both qi and Yin leading to collapse, myocardial infarction, cardiogenic shock, septic shock, etc.	1. Intramuscular injection: 2–4 ml once, 1–2 times a day. 2. Intravenous drip: 20–60 ml, diluted with 250–500 ml 5% glucose injection, or as directed by the doctor.	1. This product is not suitable for patients with chest pain caused by cold coagulation and blood stasis. It is forbidden for newborns and infants; it is forbidden to use it for those who are still suffering from heat evil such as excess syndrome or summer heat disease, and those whose symptoms are not solved due to cough; it should be used with caution for pregnant women and patients with drug allergy history or allergic constitution. Clinical monitoring should be strengthened for the elderly and the weak and the patients with severe cardiopulmonary diseases. 2. This product should not be used together with traditional Chinese medicine containing Veratrum, wulingzhi, and other Western medicines.

| 7. | Shenfu Injection | In each bottle 10 ml | Restoring yang and rescuing patient from collapse, invigorating qi for consolidating superficies. It can also be used for palpitation, cough, stomachache, diarrhea, arthralgia caused by Yang deficiency or qi deficiency. | 1. Intramuscular injection: 2–4 ml once, 1–2 times a day.
2. Intravenous drip: 20–100 ml once (with 5–10% glucose injection) 250–500 ml, diluted and used).
3. Intravenous injection: 5–20 ml once (diluted with 20 ml of 5–10% glucose injection), or according to the doctor's advice. | 1. This product contains aconite (heishun tablet), which should be used strictly according to the doctor's advice.
2. It is forbidden to use this product in case of allergy or history of serious adverse reactions; it is forbidden for newborns and infants. It is not suitable for excess heat syndrome and yin deficiency syndrome.
3. It should not be used with drugs containing Pinellia ternate, Trichosanthes kirilowii, Rhizoma Fritillariae, Rhizoma Atractylodis, and Veratrum.
4. The drug should be used in strict accordance with the functional indications specified in the drug instructions, and off-label use is prohibited. Strictly control the usage and dosage, strictly prohibit the mixture and compatibility, and carefully combine the drugs. |

3. The drug should be used in strict accordance with the functional indications specified in the drug instructions, and off-label use is prohibited. Strictly control the usage and dosage, strictly prohibit mixing and compatibility, and be cautious of combined medication.

(Continued)

Table 1. (*Continued*)

Serial number	Name of drug	Specifications	Functional indications	Usage and dosage	Matters needing attention
8.	Shenmai Injection	In each bottle 10 ml	Invigorating qi for consolidating superficies, nourishing yin and promoting the production of body fluid, increasing heart rate. It is used to treat shock, coronary heart disease, viral myocarditis, chronic pulmonary heart disease, and granulocytopenia. It can improve the immune function of tumor patients. When combined with chemotherapy drugs, it has a certain synergistic effect and can reduce the side effects caused by chemotherapy drugs.	1. Intramuscular injection: 2–4 ml once a day. 2. Intravenous drip: 20–100 ml at a time (diluted with 250–500 ml 5% glucose injection, or by direct drip); or as directed by the doctor.	1. It is forbidden to use this product in case of allergy or history of serious adverse reactions; it is forbidden for newborns and infants. Pregnant women, the elderly, and weak; patients with serious cardiopulmonary disease should use with caution, and clinical monitoring should be strengthened when using drugs. 2. It is not suitable for compatibility with traditional Chinese medicine containing Veratrum and wulingzhi and Western medicine that reacts with the drug. 3. The daily dosage should not be less than 200 ml when it is used to rescue critically ill patients. If the dosage is too small, it may affect the curative effect. 4. The drug should be used in strict accordance with the functional indications specified in the drug instructions, and off-label use is prohibited. Strictly control the usage and dosage, strictly prohibit the mixture and compatibility, and carefully combine the drugs.

Appendix

1. Qingfei Paidu Decoction (Lung-Cleansing and Detoxifying Decoction)

Source of prescription: Notice of the General Office of the National Health Commission and the state administration of traditional Chinese medicine Office on Recommending the Use of "Qingfei Paidu Decoction" **(Lung-Cleansing and Detoxifying Decoction)** in Treating Pneumonia Infected by novel coronavirus with Integrated Traditional Chinese and Western Medicine (No. 22 [2020] of the State Administration of Traditional Chinese Medicine).

Ingredients: Ephedra (*Herba Ephedrae.*) 9 g, Liquorice Root (*Radix Glycyrrhizae.*) 6 g, Bitter Almond (*Armeniacae Amarum Semen.*) 9 g, Raw Gypsum (*Gypsum Fibrosum.*) 15–30 g (decocted first), Ramulus Cinnamomi (*Cassia Twig.*) 9 g, Rhizoma Alismatis (*Oriental Waterplantain Rhizome.*) 9 g, Agaric (*Polyporus.*) 9 g, Largehead Atractylodes Rhizome (*Rhizoma Atractylodis Macrocephalae.*) 9 g, Indian Buead (*Poria.*) 15 g, Chinese Thorowax Root (*Radix Bupleuri.*) 16 g, Baical Skullcap Root (*Radix Scutellariae.*) 6 g, Pinellia Tuber (*Rhizome Pinelliae.*) 9 g, Ginger (*Radix Scutellariae.*) 9 g, Tatarian Aster Root (*Radix Asteris.*) 9 g, winter flower (*Flos Farfarae.*) 9 g, Blackberrykiky Rhizome (*Rhizoma Bela-mcandae.*) 9 g, Manchurian Wildginger (*Herba Asari.*) 6 g, Common Yam Rhizome (*Rhizoma Diosscoreae.*) 12 g, Immature Bitter Orange (*Fructus Aurantii Immaturus.*) 6 g, Tangerine Peel (*Pericarpium Citri Reticulatae.*) 6 g, and Wrinkled Gianthyssop Herb (*Herba Agastaches.*) 9 g.

Indication: This decoction can be used in the treatment of mild, moderate, severe, and critical patients based on the actual situation of the individuals.

Administration: Decocting in water for oral administration. One dose per day, one serving both in the morning and in the evening (40 minutes after the meal), take it when it is warm; three doses for one course of treatment.

2. Huashi Baidu Granules (Dampness-Resolving and Detoxifying Granules)

Source of prescription: Chinese Academy of Chinese Medical Sciences.

Ingredients: Ephedra (*Herba Ephedrae.*) 6 g, Bitter Apricot Seed (*Semen Armeniacae Amarum.*) 9 g, Gypsum (*Gypsum Fibrosum.*) 15 g (decocted first), Liquorice Root (*Radix Glycyrrhizae.*) 3 g, Wrinkled Gianthyssop Herb (*Herba Agastaches.*) 10 g (decocted later), Officinal Magnolia Bark (*Cortex Magnoliae Officinalis.*) 10 g, Swordlike Atractylodes Rhizome (*Rhizoma Atractylodis.*) 15 g, Tsaoko Amomum Fruit (*Fructus Tsaoko.*) 10 g, processed Pinellia tuber (*Rhizoma Pinelliae.*) 9 g, Indian Buead (*Poria.*) 15 g, Rhubarb (*Radix et Rhizoma Rhei.*) 5 g (decocted late.), Membranous Milkvetch Root (*Radix Astragali.*) 10 g, Pepperweed Seed (*Semen Lepidii.*) 10 g, and Red Paeony Root (*Radix Paeoniae Rubra.*) 10 g.

Indication: Severe cases with syndrome of lung blocking due to epidemic toxin.

Administration: 1–2 doses per day, decocted in water, 100–200 ml each time, 2–4 times a day, oral or nasal administration.

3. Xuanfei Baidu Tang (Lung-Ventilating and Detoxifying Decoction)

Source of prescription: Wuhan Hospital of Traditional Chinese Medicine and Hubei Hospital of Integrated Traditional Chinese and Western Medicine.

Ingredients: Ephedra (*Herba Ephedrae.*) 6 g, Bitter Apricot Seed (*Semen Armeniacae Amarum.*) 15 g, Gypsum (*Gypsum Fibrosum.*) (decocted first) 30 g, raw Coix Seed (*Semen Coicis.*) 30 g, Swordlike Atractylodes Rhizome (*Rhizoma Atractylodis.*) 10 g, Cablin Potchouli Herb (*Herba

Pogostemonis.) 15 g, Sweet Wormwood Herb (*Herba Artemisiae.*) 12 g (decocted later), Giant Knotweed Rhizome (*Rhizoma Polygoni Cuspidati.*) 20 g, European Verbena (*Herba Verbenae.*) 30 g, dried Reed Rhizome (*Rhizoma Phragmitis.*) 30 g, Pepperweed Seed (*Semen Lepidii.*) 15 g, Pummelo Peel (*Exocarpium Citri Grandis.*) 15 g, and raw Liquorice Root (*Radix Glycyrrhizae.*) 10 g.

Indication: Mild and moderate cases.

4. NO. 1 Prescription Recommended by Guangdong Province

Source of prescription: Notice of Guangdong Provincial Drug Administration, Health Commission of Guangdong Province and Guangdong Provincial Administration of Traditional Chinese Medicine on Relevant Provisions for Clinical Use of Toujie Quwen Granules (formerly known as "Pneumonia No. 1 Prescription") (Permit No. 8 [2020] of Guangdong Food and Drug Administration).

Ingredients: Weeping forsythia capsule (*Fructus Forsythiae.*), common pleione pseudobulb (*Pseudobulbus Cremastrae seu Pleiones.*), lonicera japonica (*Flos Lonicerae.*), scutellaria baicalensis (*Radix Scutellariae.*), bupleurum (*Bupleurum chinense.*), sweet wormwood herb (*Herba Artemisiae Annuae.*), cicada slough (*Periostracum Cicadae.*), Hogfennel Root (*Radix Peucedani.*), fritillary bulb (*Fritillaria.*), dark plum (*Fructus Mume.*), scrophularia ningpoensis (*Radix Scrophulariae.*), ground beetle (*Eupolyphaga Seu Steleophaga.*), atractylodes rhizome (*Rhizoma Atractylodis.*), astragalus mongholicus (*Radix Astragali seu Hedysari.*), heterophylly falsestarwort root (*Radix Pseudostellariae.*), and poria cocos (*Poria.*).

Indication: Mild cases.

5. NO. 2 Prescription Recommended by Guangdong Province

Source of prescription: "Notice on Printing and Distributing the Treatment Plan of Traditional Chinese Medicine in novel coronavirus, Guangdong Province" (Trial Second Edition) (Guangdong Traditional

Chinese Medicine Office [2020] Mandate No. 31) issued by Guangdong Provincial Health Committee Office and Guangdong Provincial Administration of Traditional Chinese Medicine Office.

Ingredients: Sun-dried ginseng (*Radix Ginseng.*) 10 g (decocted separately), fried atractylodes (*Rhizoma Atractylodis Macrocephalae.*) 15 g, poria cocos (Poria.) 15 g, white hyacinth bean (*Semen Dolichoris Album.*) 30 g, lotus seed (*Semen Nelumbinis.*) 15 g, yam (*Dioscorea oppositifolia L.*) 15 g, coix seed (*Semen Coicis.*) 30 g, amomum villosum (*Fructus Amomi Villosi.*) 5 g (decocted later), platycodon grandiflorum (*Radix Platycodonis*) 10 g, roasted malt (Fructus Hordei Germinatus.) 30 g, medicated leaven (*Massa Medicata Fermentata.*) 10 g, and honey-fried licorice root (*Glycyrrhiza uralensis Fisch.*) 5 g.

Indication: Convalescent patients with deficiency of both the lungs and spleen.

6. NO. 1 Prescription Recommended by Hubei Province — Qingfei dayuan granules (formerly known as "pneumonia No. 1")

Source of prescription: Hubei Provincial Hospital of Traditional Chinese Medicine.

Ingredients: Bupleurum root (*Bupleurum Falcatum*) 20 g, scutellaria root (*Scutellaria baicalensis*) 10 g, Pinellia tuber (*Pinellia*) 10 g, codonopsis pilosula (*Codonopsis*) 15 g, whole melon withering (*Totum cucumis*) 10g, areca nut (*Betel Nucis*) 10 g, amomum tsao-ko (*Tsaoko*) 15 g, magnolia officinalis (*Magnolia grandiflora*) 15 g, anemarrhena rhizome (*Mater*) 10 g, peony (*Paeonia lactiflora*) 10 g, raw licorice (*Rudis Licoricia*) 10 g, tangerine peel (*Cort*) 10 g, and giant knotweed rhizome (*Knotweed*) 10 g.

Indication: Patients with Dampness Syndrome of Shaoyang in the Early Stage.

Administration: 1 dose per day, decocted in water, taken 3 times, one time in the morning, one time in the middle, and one time in the evening. Take it before meals.

7. NO. 2 Prescription Recommended by Hubei Province — Pneumonia Prescription 2

Source of prescription: Hubei Provincial Hospital of Traditional Chinese Medicine.

Ingredients: Ephedra (*Ephedra*) 10 g, almond (*Semen Armeniacae Amarum*) 10 g, coix seed (*CoixSemen*) 30 g, coptis root (*Coptis*) 6 g and Pinellia tuber (*Pinellia*) 10 g, snakegourd peel (*Snakegourd Peel*) 10 g, amomum tsao-ko (*Tsaoko*) 10 g, Rhizoma anemarrhenae (*Mater*) 10 g, cordate houttuynia (*Houttuynia Aucuparia*) 15 g, raw liquorice (*Rudis Licoricia*) 10 g, and round cardamom fruit 10 g (*Alba Amomum*).

Indication: Patients with dampness-heat and lung stagnation syndrome.

8. Prescription NO. 1 Recommended by Zhejiang Province

Prescription Source: Zhejiang Administration of Traditional Chinese Medicine "Zhejiang Provincial Recommendations for Prevention and Control of Novel Coronavirus Pneumonia by Traditional Chinese Medicine" (Trial Fourth Edition).

Ingredients: Herba Schizonepetae (*Nepeta*) 10 g, Radix Saposhnikoviae (*Windproof*) 10 g, Notopterygii Rhizoma (*Rhizoma et Radix Notopterygii*) 10 g, Folium Perillae (*Su vobis*) 10 g, Rhizoma Atractylodis (*Rhizoma Atractylodis*) 12 g, pericarpium citri reticulatae (*Cort*) 10 g, magnolia officinalis (*Magnolia grandiflora*) 10 g, amomum tsao-ko (*Tsaoko*) 6 g, lithospermum (*Lithospermum erythrorhizon*) 15 g, forsythia (*Forsythia*) 15 g, belamcanda rhizome (*Offa Aridam*) 9 g, cyrtomium fortunei (*Cyrtomium Fortunei*) 10g, and agastache rugosa (*Ageratum*) 10 g.

Indication: Mild cases with syndrome of the lungs invaded by epidemic toxin.

9. Prescription NO. 2 Recommended by Zhejiang Province

Prescription Source: Zhejiang Administration of Traditional Chinese Medicine "Zhejiang Provincial Recommendations for Prevention and

Control of Novel Coronavirus Pneumonia by Traditional Chinese Medicine" (Trial Fourth Edition).

Ingredients: Semen lepidii (*Semen Lepidii*) 15 g, pericarpium trichosanthis (*Pericarpium Trichosanthis*) 9 g, wild buckwheat root (*Buckwheat radix feram*) 30 g, lung-shaped grass (*Pulmonis-herba Informibus*) 30 g, parched Scutellaria baicalensis Georgi (*Scutellaria Fricta*) 30 g, Perilla frutescens (*Perilla Frutescens*) 9 g, Allium macrostemon Bunge (*Scallion*) 12 g, ginger processed pinellia (*Jiang Pinxia*) 12 g, cassia twig (*Cassia Twig*) 9 g, raw white paeony root (*Paeonia lactiflora Pall*) 15 g, Chuanxiong rhizome (*Chuanxiong Rhizome*) 15 g, and white mustard seed (*Alba*) 9 g.

Indication: Severe cases with the syndrome of epidemic toxin obstructing the lungs.

10. Prescription NO. 1 Recommended by Ningxia Hui Autonomous Region

Prescription Source: Ningxia Hui Autonomous Region Administration of Traditional Chinese Medicine "Ningxia Provincial Recommendations for Prevention and Control of Novel Coronavirus Pneumonia by Traditional Chinese Medicine" (Trial).

Ingredients: Fried Rhizoma atractylodis (*Atractylodes Fricta*) 15 g, dried orange peel (*Cort*) 10 g, ginger magnolia bark (*Magnolia officinalis Rehd. et Wils.*) 10 g, of patchouli (*Patchouli*) 10 g and tsaoko (*Tsaoko*) 6 g, raw ephedra (*Rudis Ephedra*) 6 g, notopterygium root (*Rhizoma et Radix Notopterygii*) 10 g, ginger (*Gingiberi*) 10 g, and fried betel nut (*Betel Nucis Frixum*) 10 g.

Indication: Clinical treatment for patients with the syndrome of cold-dampness stagnation of the lungs in the initial stage. Clinical manifestations are aversion to cold, fever or no fever, dry cough, dry throat, lassitude, chest tightness, epigastric fullness or vomiting, loose stool, pale or pale red tongue, white and greasy fur, and moist pulse.

Administration: 5 doses, 1 dose per day, decocted in water.

11. Prescription NO. 1 Recommended by Ningxia Hui Autonomous Region

Prescription Source: Ningxia Hui Autonomous Region Administration of Traditional Chinese Medicine "Ningxia Provincial Recommendations for Prevention and Control of Novel Coronavirus Pneumonia by Traditional Chinese Medicine" (Trial).

Ingredients: Bitter almond (*Amarae Nuces Adiectae*) 10 g, gypsum (*Gipsum*) 30 g (decocted first), snakegourd (*Snakegourd*) 30 g, rhubarb (*Rheum. Officinale Baill*) 6 g (decocted later), main ephedra (*Ephedra*) 6 g, of ephedra (*Rudis Ephedra*) 6 g, semen lepidii (*Semen Lepidii*) 10 g, peach kernel (*Persici Gunt Nucleum Fricta*) 10 g, betel nut (*Betel Nucis Frixum*) 10 g, amomum tsao-ko (*Tsaoko*) 6 g, and atractylodes rhizome (*Atractylodes Fricta*) 10 g.

Indication: Clinical treatment of patients with the syndrome of lung closure due to epidemic toxin in the middle stage. The clinical manifestation is fever that does not subdue. Cough with little or yellow sputum, abdominal distention and constipation, chest tightness and shortness of breath, cough and dyspnea, panting when moving, and red tongue, yellow and greasy or yellow and dry coating, smooth and rapid pulse.

Administration: 5 doses, 1 dose per day, decocted in water.

Bibliography

[1] Wenzhong Zhang. Novel coronavirus pneumonia pre hospital medical emergency prevention and control manual. Beijing: Science Press, 2020.

[2] Qi Wang, Xiaohong Gu, Qingquan Liu. Novel coronavirus pneumonia Handbook of Chinese medicine diagnosis and treatment. Beijing: China Press of Traditional Chinese Medicine, 2020.

[3] Yipin Fan, Yanping Wang, Huamin Zhang, etc. Analysis of treating novel coronavirus (2019-nCoV) pneumonia from cold epidemic disease. *Journal of Traditional Chinese Medicine*, 2020, 61(5): 369–374.

[4] Min Gu, Jiao Liu, Nannan Shi, etc. Analysis of Medicine efficacy of novel coronavirus pneumonitis by TCM staging. *China Journal of Chinese Materia Medica*, 2020, 45(6): 1253 1258.

[5] Jiaju Ma, Fei Pan, Yuguang Wang. Textual research on the origin and treatment of damp disease prescriptions. *World Journal of Integrated Traditional and Western Medicine*, 2020, 15(2): 197–202.

[6] Shufeng Xiao. The pharmacological action and clinical application of Huoxiang Zhengqi pill. *Chinese Medicine Modern Distance Education of China*, 2014, 12(6): 100.

[7] Zhixin Fang. Pharmacology and clinical study of Huoxiang Zhengqi prescription in the prevention and treatment of gastrointestinal diseases. *Journal of Changchun University of Traditional Chinese Medicine*, 2013, 29(4): 726–728.

[8] Xiongfei Zhang. Progress in pharmacology and clinical research of Huoxiang Zhengqi powder. *Contemporary Medicine (Academic)*, 2008(5): 137–139.

[9] Shanxi Huayuan Pharmaceutical Biotechnology Co., Ltd. Instructions for Huoxiang Zhengqi Capsule. Drug Approval Number: Chinese Medicine Standard Character: Z20003369, 2014-12-26.

[10] Tianshili Pharmaceutical Group Co., Ltd. Instructions for use of Huoxiang Zhengqi (dropping) pill. Drug Approval Number: Chinese Medicine Standard Character: Z20000048, 2018-03-16.

[11] Hunan Hansen Pharmaceutical Co., Ltd. Instructions for use of Huoxiang Zhengqi (watered) pill. Drug Approval Number: Chinese Medicine Standard Character: Z43020884, 2008-07-23.

[12] Wuhu zhanghengchun Pharmaceutical Co., Ltd. Instructions for use of Huoxiang Zhengqi (concentrated) pill. Drug Approval Number: Chinese Medicine Standard Character: Z34020136, 2015-12-01.

[13] Hebei Hengli Group Pharmaceutical Co., Ltd. Instructions for use of Huoxiang Zhengqi water. Drug Approval Number: Z13021785, 2015-12-01.

[14] Taiji Group Chongqing Fuling Pharmaceutical Factory Co., Ltd. Instructions for use of Huoxiang Zhengqi oral liquid. Drug Approval Number: Chinese Medicine Standard Character: Z50020409, 2018-03-22.

[15] Zhixin Fang, Ruili Liu, Hui Wu, *et al.* Literature analysis of clinical adverse reactions of Huoxiang Zhengqi preparation. *Henan Traditional Chinese Medicine*, 2015, 35(6): 1434–1436.

[16] Songsong Liu, Yiming Xie. Document analysis of 101 cases of adverse drug reactions of Huoxiang Zhengqi water. *Chinese Journal of Pharmacovigilance*, 2017, 14(5): 317– 320.

[17] Guangyuan Lei, Zhaobao Lei. Analysis of 101 cases of adverse reactions/ events caused by Huoxiang Zhengqi water. *Chinese Traditional Patent Medicine*, 2012, 34(11): 2268–2269.

[18] Shaojun Liu, Qingli Yang. Analysis of 80 cases of adverse reactions/events caused by Huoxiang Zhengqi water. *Contemporary Medicine*, 2014, 20(7): 133–134.

[19] Aijuan Hei. Analysis of 10 cases of convulsion in children caused by Huoxiang Zhengqi water. *Journal of Modern Medicine & Health*, 2011, 27(24): 3744.

[20] Yenan Tan, Tian Gao, Xujie Zhang, *et al.* One case of gastrointestinal bleeding caused by Huoxiang Zhengqi water. *Chinese Journal of Pharmacovigilance*, 2009, 6(12): 759–760.

[21] Tong Wang. Effect of oseltamivir phosphate assisted Huoxiang Zhengqi pill in the treatment of influenza. *Acta Medicine Sinica*, 2016, 29(1): 69–71.

[22] Jianheng Li, Xinghonog Zhang, Dayi Hou, *et al.* Effect of Huoxiang Zhengqi tablet on spontaneous activity of mice. *China Pharmaceuticals*, 2005(5): 26.

[23] Yan Ma. Analysis of Huoxiang Zhengqi oral liquid combined with norfloxacin in the treatment of AGE. *Chinese Medicine Modern Distance Education of China*, 2018, 16(8): 107–108.

[24] Bao Wei. Effect of Huoxiang Zhengqi pill combined with omeprazole enteric coated tablets on acute gastroenteritis. *Gansu Science and Technology*, 2018, 34(4): 99–100.

[25] Yin Chen, Genxi Wu, Weihua Tang. Observation on the effect of low dose erythromycin combined with Huoxiang Zhengqi water in the treatment of neonatal functional vomiting. *China Practical Medicine*, 2013, 8(36): 196–197.

[26] Changqing Shen, Yanfeng Jing. The incompatibility of Chinese patent medicine and chemical medicine in digestion. *China Practical Medicine*, 2011, 6(15): 141–142.

[27] Hongmin Cui, Hongjie Cui. Interaction between alcohol and drugs. *Journal of Binzhou Medical University*, 2003 (2): 146–147.

[28] Aogeriletu, Zhibin Xiao. Adverse reactions caused by drug alcohol inter-action. *World Lasted Medicine Information*, 2018, 18(9): 234–236.

[29] Rongfen Xia. Clinical compatibility and potential safety of traditional Chinese Medicine. *Nei Mongol Journal of Traditional Chinese Medicine*, 2012, 31(2): 55–56.

[30] Wei Lu, Wenjin Wu. Progress in pharmacological research of Huoxiang Zhengqi prescription. *Chinese Journal of Information on Traditional Chinese Medicine*, 2008(S1): 82–83.

[31] Zexiang Wang, Dan Lu, Peng Zhang, *et al.* Chemical compos-ition, pharmacological action and prediction of quality marker of Huoxiang Zhengqi formula. *China Medicine and Pharmacy*, 2019, 9(21): 28–34+59.

[32] Chunyuan Li, Xiangyu Zhou, Shengqian Wu, *et al.* The effect of Huoxiang Zhengqi oral liquid on urine metabolomics of rats with syndrome of damp-ness retaining in spleen and stomach. *Traditional Chinese Drug Research and Clinical Pharmacology*, 2017, 28(4): 499–503.

[33] Yao Liu, Wei Liu. The effect of Huoxiang Zhengqi powder on the immune and metabolic function of sub-health animal of dampness retaining in spleen and stomach. *Lishizhen Medicine and Materia Medica Research*, 2011, 22(5): 1190–1192.

[34] Lifang Sun. New clinical use and adverse reactions of pinellia tuber. *Hebei Journal of Traditional Chinese Medicine*, 2010, 32(7): 1057–1058.

[35] Wenbin Hu, Han Wang, Shaofei Zhang, *et al.* Research progress in chemical constituents, drug properties and toxicity of pinellia tuber. *China Resources Comprehensive Utilization*, 2016, 34(10): 57–59.

[36] Juxiechang (Beijing) Pharmaceutical Co., Ltd. Operation manual of Jinhua Qinggan granules. Drug Approval Number: Chinese Medicine Standard Character: Z20160001, 2016-09-02.

[37] Guoqin Li, Jing Zhao, Zhitao Tu, *et al.* Double blind randomized controlled trial of Jinhua Qinggan Granule in the treatment of influenza for wind-heart invading lung. *Chinese Journal of Integrated Traditional and Western Medicine*, 2013, 33(12): 1631–1635.

[38] Beijing Traditional Chinese Medicine. Scientific prevention and treatment of influenza A H1N1 — Record of new drug research and development of Jinhua Qinggan formula. *Beijing Journal of Traditional Chinese Medicine*, 2009, 28(12): 981.

[39] Xiaohui Dai. Analysis of adverse reactions caused by combination of traditional Chinese medicine and Western Medicine. *China Pharmacy*, 2008 (15): 1199–1200.

[40] Zhiguo Liu, Li Liu, Guoqin Li, *et al.* Randomized double-blind controlled study on the dose-response relationship of traditional Chinese medicine in the wind-heat syndrome. *Chinese Journal of Basic Medicine in Traditional Chinese Medicine*, 2013, 19(11): 1328–1330+1378.

[41] Rongfen Xia. Clinical compatibility and potential safety of traditional Chinese Medicine. *Nei Mongol Journal of Traditional Chinese Medicine*, 2012, 31(2): 55–56.

[42] Jianping Qi, Xiaoyuan Qi, Xiaojuan Wang. Effect of different doses of Jinhua Qinggan Granule on influenza and serum cytokines in patients[J]. *Modern Medical Journal*, 2016, 44(12): 1664–1669.

[43] Ling Huang, Yan Wang, Shuyue Wu. Research progress in pharmacological action of Ephedra. *China Foreign Medical Treatment*, 2018, 37(7): 195–198.

[44] Chunyan Zhang, Ruizhen Cheng, Tao Wang. Research status of the efficacy of substance basis and safety of Ephedra. *Hubei Journal of Traditional Chinese Medicine*, 2018, 40(2): 58–61.

[45] Lili Peng, Lan Li, Lu Shen, *et al.* Literature analysis of 175 cases of adverse drug reactions/events caused by Lianhuaqingwen capsule. *Chinese Journal of Pharmacovigilance*, 2015, 12(12): 753–755+759.

[46] Shiheng Wang, Jianfeng Liu, Yili Zhang, *et al.* Systematic evaluation of the efficacy and safety of Lianhuaqingwen capsule in the treatment of viral cold[J]. *China Journal of Chinese Materia Medica*, 2019, 44(7): 1503–1508.

[47] Shuo Shen, Chuangfeng Zhang, Feng Wei, *et al.* Study on the chemical constituents of Lianhuaqingwen capsule(III). *Chinese Traditional and Herbal Drugs*, 2019, 50(4): 814–820.

[48] Dan Bi, Yunbo Sun, Lianqiang Song, *et al.* Study on the chemical constituents of Lianhuaqingwen capsule(I). *Chinese Traditional and Herbal Drugs*, 2018, 49(4): 795–800.

[49] Chuangfeng Zhang, Shuo Shen, Lianqiang Song, *et al.* Study on the chemical constituents of Lianhuaqingwen capsule(II). *Chinese Traditional and Herbal Drugs*, 2018, 49(14): 3222–3225.

[50] Xue Bai. Study on the chemical constituents of Lianhuaqingwen capsule. *Capital Food Medicine*, 2019, 26(22): 187.

[51] Xifeng Gao. Study on the chemical constituents of Lianhua Qingwen capsule the analysis of the blood components of Lianhua Qingwen capsule by UPLC-Q-TOF-MS. *China Health Care Nutrition*, 2018, 28(14): 226–227.

[52] Shoujun Wang. Study on the pharmacological mechanism of Lianhu-aqingwen capsule against influenza virus. *Chinese Journal of Clinical Rational Drug Use*, 2019, 12(5): 53–54.

[53] Hai Guo, Jin Yang, Jiening Gong, *et al.* Effect of Lianhuaqingwen Capsule on lung index of mice infected with virus. *Henan Traditional Chinese Medicine*, 2007(3): 35–36.

[54] Xianghao Wen, Chong Li, Lu Guo, *et al.* Effect of Lianhuaqingwen Capsule on the proliferation inhibition and apoptosis induction of breast cancer MCF-7 cells. *Strait Pharmaceutical Journal*, 2014, 26(12): 235–238.

[55] Duan Zhong-Ping, Jia Zhen-Hua, Zhang Jian, *et al.* Natural herbal medicine Lianhuaqingwen capsule anti-influenza A (H1N1) trial: A randomized, double blind, positive controlled clinical trial. *Chin Med J (Engl)*, 2011, 124(18): 2925–33.

[56] Yuewen Ding, Lijuan Zeng, Runfeng Li, *et al.* The Chinese prescription lianhuaqingwen capsule exerts anti-influenza activity through the inhibition of viral propagation and impacts immune function. *BMC Complement Altern Med*, 2017, 17(1).

[57] Hongtao Lei, Minyan Liu, Jingfeng Ouyang, *et al.* Study on the anti Staphylococcus aureus biofilm of Lianhuaqingwen capsule. *Chinese Journal of Experimental Traditional Medical Formulae*, 2013, 19(22): 161–164.

[58] Like Shi, Yu Wang, Xing Dong, *et al.* In vitro antibacterial effect of Lianhuaqingwen combined with meropenem on resistant strains. *Chinese Journal of Nosocomiology*, 2019, 29(8): 1172–1175.

[59] Mei Wei, Yuxun Song, Hong Zhou. The effect of Lianhuaqingwen Capsule on acute upper respiratory tract infection and its effect on IFN-γ. *Chinese Journal of Difficult and Complicated Cases*, 2014, 13(4): 345–348.

[60] Lei Chen. The effect of Lianhua Qingwen Capsule on acute suppurative tonsillitis and the recovery time of body temperature. *Chinese Journal of Modern Drug Application*, 2019, 13(22): 203–204.

[61] Kunsong Dai. Clinical observation on the treatment of 56 children with acute suppurative tonsillitis with the combination of traditional Chinese and Western Medicine. *Tianjin Pharmacy*, 2019, 31(1): 35–37.

[62] Yanqing Li. Clinical application of Shufeng Jiedu Capsule. *Journal of Emergency in Traditional Chinese Medicine*, 2017, 26(4): 652–655+658.

[63] Ting Jin. Incompatibility of Danshen and ephedra preparation with Western Medicine. *Capital Medicine*, 2006(7): 31.

[64] Anhui Jiren Pharmaceutical Co., Ltd. Instructions of Shufeng Jiedu Capsule. Drug Approval Number: Chinese Medicine Standard Character: Z20090047, 2018-09-20.

[65] Xiaoyan Xu, Xianfei Li, Jing Zhang., *et al*. One case of adverse reaction caused by Shufeng Jiedu Capsule. *Chinese Journal of Pharmaco-epidemiology*, 2014, 23(11): 677.

[66] Qifu Wu. Progress in clinical application of Shufeng Jiedu Capsule in the treatment of pediatric diseases. *Journal of Emergency in Traditional Chinese Medicine*, 2017, 26(9): 1616–1618.

[67] Chunxiang Xu, Sijun He. Clinical observation of Shufeng Jiedu Capsule Combined with amoxicillin and clavulanate potassium in the treatment of acute tonsillitis. *Clinical Journal of Traditional Chinese Medicine*, 2016, 28(02): 224–226.

[68] Youliang Wei. Clinical observation of Shufeng Jiedu Capsule Combined with antibiotics in the treatment of acute exacerbation of chronic bronchitis. *China Modern Medicine*, 2019, 26(8): 55–57.

[69] Xiaoxia Liu, Jing Meng. Clinical analysis of Shufeng Jiedu Capsule Combined with acyclovir eye drops in the treatment of 100 cases of herpes simplex keratitis. *Lingnan Journal of Emergency Medicine*, 2017, 22(2): 185–186.

[70] Huiyang Chen, Xing Zhou, Yibo He, *et al*. Clinical observation of Shufeng Jiedu Capsule Combined with ciprofloxacin and vitamin C in the treatment of feifeng acne. *Drug Evaluation Research*, 2017, 40(12): 1787–1789.

[71] Yan Niu, Cao Lv, Xiaohong Yang, *et al*. Efficacy of Shufeng Jiedu Capsule Combined with antibiotics in the treatment of juvenile secretory otitis media. *Journal of Emergency in Traditional Chinese Medicine*, 2018, 27(8): 1453–1455.

[72] Ran Liu, Xuanllin Li, Liaoyao Wang, *et al*. Meta analysis and grade evaluation of Shufeng Jiedu Capsule Combined with antibiotics in the treatment of community acquired pneumonia. *Journal of Traditional Chinese Medicine*, 2018, 59(19): 1656–1660.

[73] Zhaoping Yin, Shuai Sun. Clinical study of Shufeng Jiedu Capsule Combined with levofloxacin in the treatment of acute exacerbation of chronic bronchitis. *Drugs & Clinic*, 2018, 33(11): 2880–2883.

[74] Hong Chen, Yuming Su, Jinhua Zhu. Clinical observation of Shufeng Jiedu Capsule Combined with cimetidine in the treatment of mumps in children Clinical observation of Shufeng Jiedu Capsule Combined with cimetidine in the treatment of mumps in children. *Journal of Emergency in Traditional Chinese Medicine*, 2016, 25(5): 937–938.

[75] Wenbo Zhou, Juan Rao, Ling Chen. Clinical observation of Shufeng Jiedu Capsule Combined with moxifloxacin in the treatment of community acquired pneumonia. *Journal of Emergency in Traditional Chinese Medicine*, 2019, 28(8): 1460–1462.

[76] Xia Wu, Yi Mao, Huimin Wu. Shufeng Jiedu Capsule Combined with cefoperazone sodium and sulbactam sodium in the treatment of community acquired pneumonia. *Pharmaceutical Biotechnology*, 2019, 26(5): 413–415.

[77] Shangpin Li. To explore the clinical effect of oseltamivir combined with Shufeng Jiedu Capsule in the treatment of adult influenza[J]. *Journal of North Pharmacy*, 2020, 17(1): 112–113.

[78] Ziyi Wang, Hengyu Li, Xin Gao, *et al*. Evaluation of analgesic effect of four kinds of traditional Chinese medicine against cold. *Research and Practice on Chinese Medicines*, 2019, 33(4): 58–61+66.

[79] Yanqi Han, Yanan Dong, Jun Xu, *et al*. Study on the mechanism of anti inflammation and immunoregulation of Shufeng Jiedu Capsule based on network pharmacology. *Chinese Traditional and Herbal Drugs*, 2019, 50(15): 3555–3562.

[80] Yanyan Bao, Yingjie Gao, Yujing Shi, *et al*. Study on broad spectrum antiviral effect of Shufeng Jiedu Capsule. *Journal of New Chinese Medicine*, 2019, 51(12): 5–8.

[81] Huan Qiu, Zhenxing Li, Tongna Zhu, *et al*. Experimental study on antiviral effect of Shufeng Jiedu Capsule in vivo. *Traditional Chinese Drug Research and Clinical Pharmacology*, 2014, 25(1): 14–17.

[82] Weiwei Lv, Tongna Zhu, Huan Qiu, *et al*. In vitro pharmacodynamics of Shufeng Jiedu Capsule against virus and bacteria. *Traditional Chinese Drug Research and Clinical Pharmacology*, 2013, 24(3): 234–238.

[83] Jing Liu, Li Ma, Jie Lu, *et al*. Study on the Antipyretic Mechanism of Shufeng Jiedu Capsule. *Chinese Traditional and Herbal Drugs*, 2016, 47(12): 2040–2043.

[84] Yuan Y, Liao Q, Xue M, *et al*. Shufeng jiedu capsules alleviate lipopolysaccharide-induced acute lung inflammatory injury via activation of GPR18 by verbenalin. *Cell Physiol. Biochem.*, 2018, 50(2): 629–639.

[85] Jiangxi Qingfeng Pharmaceutical Co., Ltd. Instructions for Xiyanping Injection. Drug Approval Number: Chinese Medicine Standard Character: Z20026249, 2015-09-02.

[86] Lili Liu, Xueying Zhang. Analysis of domestic literature on adverse reactions/events of Xiyanping Injection. *Chinese Journal of Pharmacoepidemiology*, 2013, 22(8): 457–459.

[87] Zhifei Wang, Yanming Xie. Adverse events of Xiyanping Injection[J]. *China Journal of Chinese Materia Medica*, 2012, 37(18): 2792–2795.

[88] Yanping Wang, Kai Jiao, Zhongfang He. Systematic evaluation of literature on adverse reactions of Xiyanping Injection. *Chinese Journal of Experimental Traditional Medical Formulae*, 2011, 17(24): 236–239.

[89] Shiqi Chen. Study on the risk assessment of clinical application of Xiyanping injection and the revision procedure of its instruction manual. Beijing University of Chinese Medicine, 2019.

[90] Xiaoling Yang, Fan Cheng, Yanhong Liu, *et al*. Study on the compatible stability of Xiyanping injection and 15 kinds of drugs. *Chinese Journal of New Drugs*, 2013, 22(20): 2374–2378.

[91] Juan Zhao, Qiming Tan. The incompatibility between Xiyanping and vitamin B6[J]. *Clinical Journal of Medical Officer*, 2007(3): 410.

[92] Weiguo Xu, Tingting Hou, Weina Ding, *et al*. Adverse reactions of Xiyanping injection and preventive measures. *Medical Information (Mid ten issue)*, 2011, 24(9): 4911–4912.

[93] Ping Chen. Analysis of the application of Xiyanping Injection[J]. *Modern Preventive Medicine*, 2010, 37(15): 3000–3001.

[94] Yanan Yang. The investigation and analysis of the safety of eight kinds of Chinese medicine injection. Tianjin Medicine University, 2014.

[95] Jun Tang. Application progress of Xiyanping injection in pediatrics[J]. *Journal of Clinical Rational Drug Use*, 2012, 5(21): 162–163.

[96] Jia, C. and Fuguo, S. Progress in clinical application of Xiyanping Injection[J]. *Journal of Huaihai Medicine*, 2018, 36(3): 378–380.

[97] Wei Wang, Guoli Dong. Clinical research progress of Xiyanping Injection. *Guide of China Medicine*, 2013, 11(18): 87–88.

[98] Yang Yu, Yan Cong, Xiaodan Quan, *et al*. Pharmacodynamics of Xiyanping for injection. *Journal of Liaoning University of Traditional Chinese Medicine*, 2009, 11(7): 198–200.

[99] Yinglan Nie, Bin Fan, Han Yan, *et al*. The effect of Xiyanping Injection on the content of cytokines in alveolar lavage fluid of rats with LPS induced acute lung injury. *Chinese Journal of Basic Medicine in Traditional Chinese Medicine*, 2012, 18(9): 976–978.

[100] Li M, Yang X, Guan C, *et al*. Andrographolide sulfonate reduces mortality in Enterovirus 71 infected mice by modulating immunity. *International immunopharmacology*, 2018, (55): 142–150.

[101] Shanghai Kaibao Pharmaceutical Co., Ltd. Drug Manual of Tanreqing Injection. Drug Approval Number: Chinese Medicine Standard Character: Z20030054, 2015-08-05.

[102] Xiaofang Yang, Zhi Dong, Xiaoqin Lu, *et al*. Analysis of 376 cases of adverse reactions of Tanreqing Injection in Chongqing. *Chinese Journal of New Drugs and Clinical Remedies*, 2015, 34(3): 239–242.

[103] Na Mei, Jinghong Wang, Jing Zhang, *et al*. Analysis of 141 cases of adverse reactions of Tanreqing Injection. *Journal of China-Japan Friendship Hospital*, 2017, 31(4): 236–238.

[104] Wentan Xu, Yalan Zhang, Change Xu. Literature analysis of 123 cases of adverse reactions of Tanreqing. *Chinese Journal of Pharmacovigilance*, 2012, 9(9): 548–549.

[105] Li Yu, Zhaojuan Qiu, Xiying Tan. Analysis of 110 cases of adverse reactions of Tanreqing Injection. *Chinese Journal of Pharmacovigilance*, 2015, 12(6): 360–362.

[106] Jing Li, Bin Wang. Literature analysis of 149 cases of adverse reactions of Tanreqing Injection. *Tianjin Pharmacy*, 2016, 28(5): 34–35+63.

[107] Binghua Wei, Qing Chen. Analysis of adverse reactions of Tanreqing Injection. *China Medical Herald*, 2011, 8(1): 134–135.

[108] Liang Wang, Feng Zhang, Wansheng Chen. Analysis of adverse events of Tanreqing Injection. *China Pharmacy*, 2019, 30(5): 694–697.

[109] Lin Wang, Shu Yan. Retrospective analysis of adverse reactions of Tanreqing Injection. *Drug Evaluation Research*, 2014, 37(4): 362–366.

[110] Ying Lan, Yan Yang, Die Hu, *et al*. Evaluation of the compatibility literature of Tanreqing Injection *in vitro*. *China Pharmaceuticals*, 2018, 27(12): 52–57.

[111] Xi Wei, Xiaolin Ouyang, Ying Xu, *et al*. Changes of compatibility of Tanreqing with common infusion and other drugs. *Journal of Pediatric Pharmacy*, 2013, 19(1): 28–32.

[112] Yusong Chen, Xiaojuan Dong, Qi Wang. Observation on the compatibility of Tanreqing and common drugs. *Chinese Remedies & Clinics*, 2010, 6(8): 635.

[113] Huanwen Zeng, Dakui Chen, Jing Li. Compatibility of Tanreqing injection with 113 kinds of clinical drugs. *China Medical Herald*, 2011, 8(12): 189–190.

[114] Yanan Yang. Investigation and Analysis on safety of eight kinds of key monitoring traditional Chinese medicine injections after marketing. Tianjin Medical University, 2014.

[115] Xianjun Feng. Safety analysis on the compatibility of Tanreqing injection with ten antibiotics commonly used in pediatrics. *Guide of China Medicine*, 2013, 11(14): 664–665.

[116] Nan Wang, Xiaojun Song, Xuejian Xie. Feasibility analysis of Tanreqing injection mixed with 25 kinds of drugs. *China Pharmaceuticals*, 2014, 23(3): 20–22.

[117] Ling Guan, Bibo Liu. Compatibility of Tanreqing injection with 113 kinds of clinical drugs. *Contemporary Medicine*, 2011, 17(21), 141–142.

[118] Yaolong Xu. New progress in research on incompatibility between Tanreqing injection and common antibiotics. *Biotech World*, 2014(4): 79–80.

[119] Liu Wei, Zhang Xiawei, Mao Bing, *et al*. Systems pharmacology-based study of Tanreqing injection in airway mucus hypersecretion. *Journal of ethnopharmacology*, 2020, 249: 112425.

[120] Yanmei Li. Pharmacological effect and clinical application of Tanreqing Injection. *World Latest Medicine Information*, 2019, 19(54): 197–198.

[121] Qin Wang, Jing Pan. Pharmacological action and clinical application of Tanreqing Injection. *Medical Journal of National Defending Forces in North China*, 2010, 22(1): 41–43.

[122] Hongfeng Han, Ximing Lu. Pharmacology and clinic of Tanreqing Injection. *Journal of Henan University of Science & Technology (Medical Science)*, 2006(1): 78–79.

[123] Yanshu Pan, Na Zhang, Xiaolei Zhu, *et al*. Study on the correlation between Tanreqing injection and the pathological process of endotoxemia. *Chinese Journal of Basic Medicine in Traditional Chinese Medicine*, 2005, 11(7): 508–510.

[124] Hongyao Ren, Weiguo Liu, Xiaoling Song, *et al*. Research progress of Tanreqing Injection. *Journal of Pharmaceutical Research*, 2018, 37(12): 715–717.

[125] Tianjin, HongRi Pharmaceutical Co., Ltd. Instructions for Xuebijing Injection. Drug Approval Number: Chinese Medicine Standard Character: Z20040033, 2016-03-11.

[126] Airui Nie, Zhongkun Guo, Yu Zhang, *et al*. Literature analysis of 211 cases of adverse reactions of Xuebijing Injection. *Strait Pharmaceutical Journal*, 2019, 31(11): 246–249.

[127] Yeqing Zhao. 34 cases of adverse drug reactions of Xuebijing Injection. *Journal of Clinical Rational Drug Use*, 2018, 8(11): 86–87.

[128] Jian Fang. Analysis of adverse drug reactions of Xuebijing Injection. *Strait Pharmaceutical Journal*, 2012, 24(5): 277–278.

[129] Zheng Rui, Wang Hui, Liu Zhi, *et al*. A real-world study on adverse drug reactions to Xuebijing injection: Hospital intensive monitoring based on 93 hospitals (31, 913 cases). *Annals of translational medicine*, 2019, 7(6): 117.

[130] Rongguang Qu, Jie Gao. Clinical application and evaluation of Xuebijing Injection. *Guide of China Medicine*, 2012, 10(31): 598–600.

[131] Qinglian Song, Meng Xu, Hui Yang, *et al*. Analysis of rational use of Xuebijing injection in 162 cases. *Qinghai Medical Journal*, 2015, 45(10): 65–66.

[132] Xiuqin Zeng, Aizhong Ru, Jing Liu. Investigation on the use of Xuebijing injection in inpatients. *Gansu Science and Technology*, 2018, 34(15): 145–148.

[133] Qian Hu, Guoli Yan, Congguang Wei, *et al*. Clinical application of Xuebijing injection based on the real world of his system in hospital. *Henan University of Chinese Medicine*, 2018, 38(8): 1263–1266.

[134] Shengchuan Gao, Tongchao Wang. Study on the stability of the compatibility of Xuebijing injection with various solvents. *Chinese Journal of Pharmacovigilance*, 2016, 13(3): 180–182.

[135] Xiaomei Ma, Hong Liu, Qingfang Gao. The effect of Xuebijing on the inflammatory response of endotoxin induced acute lung injury in rats. *Chinese Remedies & Clinics*, 2010, 10(5): 526–528+606.

[136] Lujun Li, Rong Ma, Yue Cao. Research progress in the mechanism of Xuebijing injection in the treatment of sepsis. *Drug Evaluation Research*, 2018, 41(8): 1548–1553.

[137] Junde Hou, Zixian Song, Yuxiang Zhang, *et al*. The effect of Xuebijing on MMP-9 level in sepsis rats and its protective effect on lung. *Hebei Medical Journal*, 2016, 36(5): 645–647.

[138] Liu Ming-Wei, Wang Yun-Hui, Qian Chuan-Yun, *et al*. Xuebijing exerts protective effects on lung permeability leakage and lung injury by upregulating Toll-interacting protein expression in rats with sepsis. *International Journal of Molecular Medicine*, 2014, 34(6): 1492–1504.

[139] Jiang Yu, Zou Lianhong, Liu Sulai, *et al*. GC/MS-based metabonomics approach reveals effects of Xuebijing injection in CLP induced septic rats. *Biomedicine & pharmacotherapy*, 2019, 117: 109163.

[140] Xu Zhaojun, Liu Danwei, Li Kairui, *et al*. To explore the preventive and therapeutic effects of Xuebijing injection on acute lung injury induced by cardiopulmonary bypass in rats by regulating the expression of micro-RNA-17-5p and its mechanism. *Zhonghua wei zhong bing ji jiu yi xue*, 2019, 31(7): 867–872.

[141] Juan Chen, Chenhuan She, Ye Zhou. Research Progress on the stability of solvent selection in finished injection of traditional Chinese Medicine. *Journal of Clinical Rational Drug Use*, 2020, 13(1): 175–177.

[142] Wuxi jiminxin Shanhe Pharmaceutical Co., Ltd. Drug Manual of Xingnaojing Injection. Drug Approval Number: Chinese Medicine Standard Character: Z32020563, Z32020564, 2010-09-30.

[143] Dali Pharmaceutical Co., Ltd. Drug Manual of Xingnaojing Injection. Drug Approval Number: Z53021638, Z53021639, Z53021640, 2010-09-20.

[144] Hongming Liu, Lili Xu, Ran Cui, *et al*. Literature analysis of 66 cases of adverse reactions of Xingnaojing Injection. *Chinese Journal of Pharmacovigilance*, 2016, 13(2): 107–110.

[145] Xiaoyan Wang, Wen Zhou, Yichi Zhang, *et al*. Analysis of adverse drug reactions caused by intravenous drip of Xingnaojing Injection in Qilu children's Hospital. *Chinese Pharmaceutical Affairs*, 2018, 32(9): 1301–1308.

[146] Zhenlei Zhou, Le Yang, Xiaoxin Guo. Analysis of 30 cases of adverse reactions/events of Xingnaojing Injection. *Chinese Journal of Pharmacovigilance*, 2014, 11(11): 683–686.

[147] Yi Yan, Li Chun-Ying, Zhao Yong, *et al*. Preclinical study on adverse reactions of Xingnaojing injection. *China journal of Chinese materia medica*, 2018, 43(13): 2789–2795.

[148] Yuan Chen, Guangming Pei. Comparative observation on insoluble particles of Xingnaojing injection with different dilutions. *Hubei Journal of Traditional Chinese Medicine*, 2016, 38(3): 72–74.

[149] Junda Xie. Literature analysis of 15 cases of adverse drug reactions caused by Xingnaojing Injection. *China Pharmacist*, 2007(9): 902–904.

[150] Linna Wu, Yun Li, Li Liu. Incompatibility between Losec injection and Xingnaojing Injection. *Chinese Journal of Practical Nursing*, 2012, 28(23): 1672–7088.

[151] Xiulu Yang, Weiyi Xu, Yuexin Gong, *et al*. Study on the pharmacological action of Xingnaojing Injection. *China Pharmacy*, 1993(1): 22–23.

[152] Junfang Li. Pharmacological analysis of Xingnaojing Injection. *China Journal of Pharmaceutical Economics*, 2014, 9(1): 48–49.

[153] Yuanhu Xu. Pharmacodynamic study and clinical application of Xingnaojing Injection. *Modern Journal of Integrated Traditional Chinese and Western Medicine*, 2010, 19(4): 507–510.

[154] Zhao Mingyi, Zhu Ping, Fujino Masayuki, *et al*. Oxidative stress in hypoxic-ischemic encephalopathy: Molecular mechanisms and therapeutic strategies. *International journal of molecular sciences*, 2016, 17(12).

[155] Jiangsu Kangyuan Pharmaceutical Co., Ltd. Instructions for Reduning Injection. Drug Approval Number: Chinese Medicine Standard Character: Z20050217, 2015-05-21.

[156] Zheng Cao, Xiangkui Shi, Jing Zhang, *et al.* Analysis of the related factors of adverse reaction report caused by Reduning Injection in 73 children with bronchopneumonia. *Anti-Infection Pharmacy*, 2019, 16(3): 476–479.

[157] Jing Chen, Beibei Chen. Analysis of 66 cases of adverse reactions of Reduning Injection. World Latest Medicine Information, 2017, 17(A4): 193–194.

[158] Danyu Kang, Ting Geng, Gang Ding, *et al.* Research progress of clinical combination and drug interaction of Reduning Injection. *China Pharmacy*, 2017, 28(2): 276–279.

[159] Feng Li, Lina Lai, Yongling Mo, *et al.* Analysis of 30 cases of adverse reactions of Reduning Injection. *Chinese Journal of Ethnomedicine and Ethnopharmacy*, 2019, 28(15): 120–122.

[160] Xiangkui Shi, Dongshen Ji, Xin Ma. Study on the stability of the compatibility of Reduning injection and ceftriaxone sodium. *Anti-Infection Pharmacy*, 2019, 16(3): 379–381+388.

[161] Yuan Li. Analysis on incompatibility of clinical drugs of Reduning Injection. *China Pharmaceuticals*, 2014, 23(19): 71–73.

[162] Zhike Yan. To explore the prevention method of adverse reactions in the combination of Reduning injection and penicillin injection. *Journal of clinical medical literature*, 2019, 6(1): 168+170.

[163] Ying Zhao. Analysis of the pharmacological action, clinical application and adverse reactions of Reduning Injection. *The Journal of Medical Theory and Practice*, 2018, 31(23): 3591–3592.

[164] Caiwen Yao. The pharmacological action, clinical application and adverse reaction analysis of Reduning Injection. *Chinese ENT News and Reviews (Otorhinolaryngology)*, 2017, 32(5): 256-257+264.

[165] Suyun Wang, Gang Li. Clinical application of Reduning Injection in pediatrics. *Global Chinese Medicine*, 2015, 8(S1): 100.

[166] Liu Jianling, Sun Ke, Zheng Chunli, *et al.* Pathway as a pharmacological target for herbal medicines: An investigation from reduning injection. *PloS One*, 2015, 10(4).

[167] Cao Zeyu, Chang Xiujuan, Zhao Zhongpeng, *et al.* Antiviral effects of Reduning injection against Enterovirus 71 and possible mechanisms of action. *Chinese Journal of Natural Medicines*, 2015, 13(12): 881–888.

[168] Lu-ping Tang, Wei Xiao, Yi-fang Li, *et al.* Anti-inflammatory effects of Reduning Injection on lipopolysaccharide-induced acute lung injury of rats. *Chinese Journal of Integrative Medicine*, 2014, 20(8): 591–599.

[169] Juan Chen, Chenhuan Yu, Ye Zhou. Research Progress on the stability of solvent selection in finished injection of traditional Chinese Medicine. *Journal of Clinical Rational Drug Use*,2020,13(1): 175–174.

[170] Ya'an Sanjiu Pharmaceutical Co., Ltd. Instructions for Shengmai Injection. Drug Approval Number: Chinese Medicine Standard Character: Z51021921, 2015-12-09.

[171] Dongyun Wang. Analysis of adverse reactions of Shengmai Injection in Taizhou City. *Strait Pharmaceutical Journal*, 2017, 29(4): 243–245.

[172] Danhua Ma, Rong Xi, Jun Sun. Characteristics and influencing factors of adverse reactions of Shengmai Injection. *Pharmaceutical and Clinical Research*, 2016, 24(4): 324–327.

[173] Peifen Huang. Clinical application and adverse reactions of Shengmai Injection. *Chinese Journal of Ethnomedicine and Ethnopharmacy*, 2015, 24(6): 97–98.

[174] Guowei Jiang, Qingqing Yi, Yongjun Meng. Serious adverse reactions of Shengmai injection: An analysis of one case. *Journal of Modern Medicine & Health*, 2015, 31(2): 319–320.

[175] Wenbin Jiao. Adverse reactions of Shengmai injection and its causes. *Contemporary Medicine Forum*, 2015, 12(5): 253.

[176] Jinhui Guo, Weifang Gao, Sujie Jia. Meta analysis of adverse reactions of Shengmai Injection. *Pharmacology and Clinics of Chinese Materia Medica*, 2013, 29(6): 168–171.

[177] Hong Zhao, Jiancheng Li. Adverse reactions of Shengmai Injection. *Chinese Journal of Drug Abuse Prevention and Treatment*, 2013, 19(6): 368–369.

[178] Jianxun Chang, Shilong Fu. Retrospective analysis of adverse reactions of Shengmai Injection. *Western Journal of Traditional Chinese Medicine*, 2013, 26(6): 48–50.

[179] Chu Tu. Literature analysis of 38 cases of adverse reactions of Shengmai Injection. *Strait Pharmaceutical Journal*, 2018, 30(4): 266–268.

[180] Juan Chen, Jun Ni, Yanyan Wang. Summary of clinical adverse reactions of Shengmai Injection. *China Reflexology*, 2017, 26(18): 120–121.

[181] Jun Feng, Jiawei Cao, Jun Yao, *et al*. Study on the compatible stability of Shengmai injection and common infusion. *Zhejiang Journal of Integrated Traditional Chinese and Western Medicine*, 2016, 26(1): 82–84.

[182] Baogang Yang, Qingkai Wang, Guangli Yin. 40 Cases of ischemic heart disease and heart failure treated with Shengmai injection and nitroprusside sodium. *Journal of Clinical Medical Literature (ElectronicEdition)*, 2018, 5(15): 37–38.

[183] Lifang Wu, Jianfeng Du. Effect of Xingnaojing combined with Shengmai Injection on expression of CD62P and inflammatory factors in patients with cerebral hemorrhage and its clinical effect. *Journal of International Neurology and Neurosurgery*, 2016, 43(3): 215–218.

[184] Jie Yang, Xiuwen Su. Puerarin Combined with Shengmai Injection in the treatment of 60 cases of coronary heart disease and heart failure. *Guide of China Medicine*, 2011, 9(29): 153–154.

[185] Yashu Fu. Effect of Shengmai injection combined with Aminophylline Injection in the treatment of 60 cases of bradyarrhythmia. *Contemporary Medicine*, 2009, 15(21): 153.

[186] Yurong Ma, Qunfen Xu. Study on the stability of the compatibility of Shengmai injection with 5% glucose injection. *China Pharmaceuticals*, 2007(14): 29.

[187] Li Hao. Study on the stability of the compatibility of Shengmai injection with 14 kinds of drugs. *Journal of Emergency in Traditional Chinese Medicine*, 2007(4): 459.

[188] Yunxia Zhao, Xiumei Wang, Maigeng Zhou. Observation on the stability of the compatibility of Shengmai injection and four kinds of intravenous injection. *Shandong Medical Journal*, 2002(32): 41–42.

[189] Qin Li, Hong Liu. Pharmacological action and clinical application of Shengmai Injection. *Medical Recapitulate*, 2005(10): 950–952.

[190] Jun Li. Pharmacological mechanism and clinical application of Shengmai Injection. *Chinese Journal of Trauma and Disability Medicine*, 2014, 22(8): 303–304.

[191] Jun Liu, Zhihong Xu. Pharmacological action and clinical application of Shengmai Injection. *Evaluation and Analysis of Drug-Use In Hospitals of China*, 2013, 13(11): 1053–1054.

[192] Xiaoming Zhang, Ya Liu. Pharmacological mechanism and clinical application of Shengmai Injection. *Medical Recapitulate*, 2013, 19(15): 2813–2816.

[193] Shuhua Xu, Shengyou Liu. Research progress in the pharmacological action of Shengmai Injection. *Chinese Pharmaceutical Affairs*, 2010, 24(4): 405–407.

[194] Cao Yan, Han Xiaotong, Pan Hongwe, *et al.* Emerging protective roles of shengmai injection in septic cardiomyopathy in mice by inducing myocardial mitochondrial autophagy via caspase-3/Beclin-1 axis. *Inflammation Research*, 2020, 69(1): 41–50.

[195] Li Yiping, Ruan Xiaofen, Xu Xiaowen, *et al.* Shengmai Injection Suppresses Angiotensin II-Induced Cardiomyocyte Hypertrophy and Apoptosis via Activation of the AMPK Signaling Pathway Through Energy-Dependent Mechanisms. *Frontiers in pharmacology*, 2019, 10: 1095.

[196] Huang Xingyue, Duan Xiaojiao, Wang Kaihuan, *et al.* Shengmai injection as an adjunctive therapy for the treatment of chronic obstructive pulmonary disease: A systematic review and meta-analysis. *Complementary therapies in medicine*, 2019, 43: 140–147.

[197] Zhang Yi, Ma Litian, Li Jie, *et al.* Anti-fibrotic Effects and Mechanism of Shengmai Injection on Human Hepatic Stellate Cells LX-2. *Chinese Journal of Integrative Medicine*, 2019, 25(3): 197–202.

[198] Zhu Jinqiang, Ye Qiaofeng, Xu Shixin, *et al.* Shengmai Injection Alleviates H2O2-induced Oxidative Stress through Activation of AKT and Inhibition of ERK Pathways in Neonatal Rat Cardiomyocytes. *Journal of Ethnopharmacology*, 2019, 239: 111677.

[199] Guangxian Zhao, Diqian Liu, Xiaolin Xin. Observation on the stability of the compatibility of Shengmai injection with four infusion solutions. *Journal of Beijing University of Traditional Chinese Medicine*, 2000(2): 43.

[200] China Resources Sanjiu (Ya'an) Pharmaceutical Co., Ltd.instructions for Shenfu Injection. Drug Approval Number: Chinese Medicine Standard Character: Z20043117, 2015-08-21.

[201] Haining Xing, Shen Li, Shuyun Li, *et al.* Analysis of adverse reactions of Shenfu Injection in 28 cases. *China Health Standard Management*, 2015, 5(10): 80–81.

[202] Zhaoxia Wu, Shilong Fu. Analysis of 130 cases of adverse reactions caused by Shenfu Injection. *China Pharmacy*, 2014, 25(16): 1496–1498.

[203] Dinjin He, Yanhong Qu. Analysis of adverse reactions of Shenfu Injection in 60 cases. *Chinese Journal of Pharmacovigilance*, 2014, 11(3): 160–162.

[204] Yingkun Fu, Yanming Xie. Clinical application and adverse reactions of Shenfu Injection. *Clinical Application and Adverse Reactions of Shenfu Injection*, 2012, 37(18): 2796–2799.

[205] Dengping Zhao, Shejun Zhang, Xuegui Jing. Observation on the effect of Shenfu Injection in the treatment of radiotherapy adverse reactions. *Seek Medical (Second Half Monthly)*, 2012, 10(9): 265.

[206] Sujuan Li. One case of adverse reaction caused by Shenfu Injection. Chinese society of Pharmacology. 2011 national pharmaceutical academic forum exchange meeting and clinical pharmacy and pharmaceutical care research progress training course proceedings. Chinese society of Pharmacology: Chinese society of Pharmacology, 2011: 259.

[207] Bin Cheng. One case of adverse reaction caused by Shenfu Injection. *Chinese Journal of Hospital Pharmacy*, 2009, 29(13): 1151.

[208] Tingqian Li, Jianxin Ma, Yudan Zhou. Clinical application and adverse reactions of Shenfu Injection. *Chinese Journal of Evidence-Based Medicine*, 2009, 9(3): 319–322.

[209] Guohua Wu, Zhaobao Lei. Analysis of 26 cases of adverse reactions caused by Shenfu Injection. *Chinese Traditional Patent Medicine*, 2015, 37(6): 1385–1387.

[210] Xueni Mo, Tiqin Liu, Yuying Hu, *et al*. Meta analysis of the efficacy and side effects of Shenfu Injection in the treatment of cardio cerebral diseases. *World Latest Medicine Information*, 2019, 19(82): 1–5.

[211] Baoping Cao, Chao Ma, Qiujiang Kuang, *et al*. Stability of compatibility of Shenfu injection and compound amino acid (18AA-VII) injection. *Chinese Journal of Medical Device*, 2017, 30(15): 1–2.

[212] Shuhua Zhang, Xiuhua Huang, Zhenrong Ou, *et al*. Study on acute toxicity of Shenfu injection combined with 12 drugs. *Journal of Emergency in Traditional Chinese Medicine*, 2005(8): 768.

[213] Shengqi Deng, Shu Chen, Jing Tao, *et al*. Study on the stability of Shenfu Injection Compatible with 12 drugs. *Journal of Emergency in Traditional Chinese Medicine*, 2005(7): 674–675.

[214] Yongdong Zhou. Stability experiment of Shenfu Injection Compatible with several infusion. *Traditional Chinese Medicinal Research*, 2002(5): 46–47.

[215] Chao Gao. Evaluation of the effect of Danshen injection and Shenfu Injection in the treatment of chronic obstructive pulmonary emphysema. *Contemporary Medicine Forum*, 2018, 16(12): 175–176.

[216] Binglin Huang. Effect of Shenfu injection combined with levosimendan on acute heart failure and its influence on inflammatory factors and brain natriuretic peptide. *Anti-Infection Pharmacy*, 2017, 14(3): 622–624.

[217] Jinbo Wu, Zhibin Wang, Cheng Yuan. The effect of erythropoietin combined with Shenfu Injection on chronic heart failure. *Chinese Journal of Evidence-Based Cardiovascular Medicine*, 2013, 5(3): 244–246.

[218] Shaogang Zhang, Jianyun Wu, Shiyan Liu, *et al*. Effect of Shenfu injection combined with meglumine cyclic adenosine on chronic congestive heart failure. *Chinese Journal of Integrative Medicine on Cardio-/Cerebrovascular Disease*, 2012, 10(4): 391–392.

[219] Shuting, D. Combined Shenfu injection and low molecular weight heparin in the treatment of heart failure in patients with severe pulmonary heart disease. *Chinese Journal of Misdiagnostics*, 2011, 11(4): 838–839.

[220] Yongbin Huang. Shenmai and Shenfu Injection in the treatment of acute myocardial infarction. *Chinese Journal of Integrated Traditional and Western Medicine in Intensive and Critical Care*, 2005(2): 107.

[221] Lihua Wang, Liqun Huang, Hongbo Lv, *et al*. The pharmacological action and clinical application of Shenfu Injection. *Medical Journal of National Defending Forces in North China*, 2010, 22(6): 535–536.

[222] Zhonghua Wang, Jinping Wang. The pharmacological action and clinical application of Shenfu Injection. *Journal of Chengde Medical College*, 2009, 26(1): 86–89.

[223] Jun Xu, Honggang Lou, Yijia Lou, *et al*. Research progress in the pharmacological action of Shenfu Injection. *Shanghai Journal of Traditional Chinese Medicine*, 2008(10): 87–89.

[224] Xuan Zhao, Chaomei Fu, Limei Cao., *et al*. Research progress of chemical components and pharmacological action of Shenfu Injection. *Pharmacy and Clinics of Chinese Materia Medica*, 2018, 9(2): 70–74.

[225] Hong Xiao. Study on the effective components of Shenfu injection and its anti cardiovascular effect. *Contemporary Medicine Forum*, 2017, 15(14): 21–22.

[226] Yuling Sui. Progress in research and clinical application of Shenfu Injection. *World Latest Medicine Information*, 2015, 15(36): 23–24.

[227] Jinqiang Zhu, Yubin Liang, Shengyu Hua, *et al*. Research progress in the components of Shenfu injection and its pharmacological effect on cardiovascular system. *Chinese Traditional Patent Medicine*, 2014, 36(4): 819–823.

[228] Xiaoheng Gao, Dayan Chen, Xiaoshuan Liu, *et al*. Research progress in pharmacological action of Shenfu Injection. *Journal of Practical Traditional Chinese Medicine*, 2013, 29(11): 972–973.

[229] Sichuan Shenghe Pharmaceutical Co., Ltd. Instructions for Shenmai Injection. Drug Approval Number: Chinese Medicine Standard Character: Z20043477, 2015-09-17.

[230] Hebei Shenwei Pharmaceutical Co., Ltd. Instructions for Shenmai Injection. Drug Approval Number: Chinese Medicine Standard Character: Z13020887, 2015-07-31.

[231] Yong Zhang. Analysis of adverse reactions caused by Shenmai Injection. *Contemporary Medicine Forum*, 2019, 17(21): 111–113.

[232] Guoying Liu. Analysis of 28 cases of adverse reactions of Shenmai Injection. *Jiangxi Medical Journal*, 2019, 54(7): 826–827.

[233] Lei Zhang. Analysis of 3 cases of adverse reactions caused by Shenmai Injection. *Chinese Journal of Drug Abuse Prevention and Treatment*, 2019, 25(1): 56–57.

[234] Baotang Liu, Yongqiang Jing, Yinfei Guo. Analysis of the influencing factors of adverse reactions of Shenmai Injection. *Hainan Medical Journal*, 2018, 29(14): 2049–2051.

[235] Fangfang He. Analysis of 154 cases of adverse reactions of Shenmai Injection. *Strait Pharmaceutical Journal*, 2018, 30(1): 271–272.

[236] Yang Liu, Longhao Xiao, Lin Li, *et al*. Literature analysis of adverse reactions of Shenmai injection in 2007–2017. Drugs & Clinic, 2017, 32(12): 2523–2528.

[237] Longyong Zeng. Analysis on the regularity and characteristics of adverse reactions of Shenmai Injection. *The Asia-pacific Traditional Medicine*, 2017, 13(21): 131–132.

[238] Mingzhao Wang, Wuqiang Qi. Clinical application and adverse reactions of Shenmai Injection. *Clinical Research and Practice*, 2017, 2(28): 102–103.

[239] Jing Xu, Yayan Zhu, Bihua Lv. Analysis of adverse reactions of Shenmai Injection. *Chinese Journal of Rural Medicine and Pharmacy*, 2017, 24(17): 31–32.

[240] Zhengbo Yan. Analysis on the combined application and adverse reactions of Shenmai Injection. *World Latest Medicine Information*, 2019, 19(91): 132–133.

[241] Jixia Fan. Application and adverse reactions of Shenmai Injection. *Journal of Clinical Rational Drug Use*, 2017, 10(35): 116–117.

[242] Zuowen Meng, Fengqin Zhai, Caili Kang. Study on the compatible Stability of Shenmai injection and common drugs. *Journal of Clinical Rational Drug Use*, 2016, 9(21): 44–45.

[243] Shenghong Yan. Study on the stability of Shenmai injection compatible with common drugs. *Healthy People*, 2014, 8(19): 14–15.

[244] Chunnong Rao, Shuijiao Liang. Study on the stability of Shenmai injection compatible with common drugs. *Pharmacy Today*, 2014, 24(1): 35–37.

[245] Yongjun Zhu, Bin Zhang. Study on the compatible stability of Shenmai injection and six common drugs. *Journal of Emergency in Traditional Chinese Medicine*, 2010, 19(10): 1742–1743.

[246] Chunying Li. Stability analysis of Shenmai injection in common drug compatibility. *Heilongjiang Medicine Journal*, 2018, 31(5): 1002–1004.

[247] Anrong Li, Xiaoqin Tian. Study on insoluble particles of Shenmai injection combined with four kinds of infusion. *China Pharmaceuticals*, 2004(6): 35–36.

[248] Li Hao. Study on the stability of Shenmai injection compatible with 14 kinds of drugs. *Journal of Emergency in Traditional Chinese Medicine*, 2007(5): 588.

[249] Xiangming Li, Shengbin Sun, Guozhi Jiang. Quality control, toxicity and clinical compatibility of Shenmai Injection. *Drug Evaluation Research*, 2019, 42(11): 2294–2300.

[250] Xiangyu Li, Li Xu. Incompatibility between Shenmai injection and Pantoprazole sodium injection. *Shandong Medical Journal*, 2010, 50(25): 46.

[251] Zhimin Tao, Suzhen Zhang, Rui Kong. The clinical pharmacological effect of Shenmai Injection on cardiovascular complications after acute myocardial infarction. *Strait Pharmaceutical Journal*, 2017, 29(4): 112–113.

[252] Jian Yu, Yanfei Xin, Yaoxian Xuan. Research progress in the material basis of Shenmai Injection. *Herald of Medicine*, 2013, 32(4): 497–500.

[253] Xiaoyang Hu. Clinical evaluation of Shenmai injection combined with Levocarnitine in the treatment of heart failure in elderly patients with ischemic cardiomyopathy. *Anti-Infection Pharmacy*, 2016, 13(5): 1166–1168.

[254] Yuxin Wen. The effect of Shenmai and compound Danshen Injection on Hemorheology in early shock patients. *Journal of Clinical Rational Drug Use*, 2016, 9(11): 37–39.

[255] Chuanjie Song. The effect of Shenmai injection combined with Levo-carnitine in the treatment of hypotension during hemodialysis. *Contemporary Medicine Forum*, 2016, 14(4): 127–128.

[256] Xiaohui Liu. Effect of Shenmai injection combined with meglumine cyclic adenosine on coronary heart disease with heart failure. *Contemporary Medicine Forum*, 2015, 13(21): 169–170.

[257] Di Wu, Jun Zhang, Xucheng Li. Effect of Shenmai injection combined with dobutamine in the treatment of cor pulmonale with acute heart failure. *Contemporary Medicine Forum*, 2015, 13(16): 175.

[258] Wenjie Dong, Jing Yu, Chengshu Miao, *et al*. Treatment of Pneumocystis carinii pneumonia with Shenmai and Huangqi Injection. *Journal of Advances in Animal Medicine*, 2015, 36(2): 124–127.

[259] Xiaomei Liu, Degang Li. Clinical observation of nitroglycerin combined with Shenmai injection in the treatment of 40 cases of heart failure. *Chinese Community Doctors*, 2013, 15(5): 207.

[260] Shengfeng Li. Effect of Shenmai injection combined with octreotide and ulinastatin on the level of inflammatory factors in patients with severe acute pancreatitis. *Contemporary Medicine Forum*, 2019, 16(1): 65–67.

[261] Xiaolong Liang, Wenhua Wang, Qingxin Shi, *et al*. Clinical observation of Shenmai injection combined with rosuvastatin calcium in the treatment of acute ischemic stroke. *Journal of New Chinese Medicine*, 2018, 50(11): 62–66.

[262] Mei Sun. Effect of Shenmai injection combined with meglumine cyclic adenosine on heart failure in patients with coronary heart disease. *Contemporary Medicine Forum*, 2018, 16(6): 80–81.

[263] Xudong Cao. Progress in pharmacological study and clinical application of Shenmai Injection. Professional Committee of traditional Chinese medicine of Zhejiang society of traditional Chinese Medicine. Proceedings of 2009 Zhejiang academic annual meeting of traditional Chinese Medicine. Professional Committee of traditional Chinese medicine of Zhejiang society of traditional Chinese Medicine: Zhejiang science and Technology Association, 2009: 164–167.

[264] Fangfang Wang, Liang Zhao, Yanjun Gao, *et al.* Pharmacological action and clinical application of Shenmai Injection. *Journal of Chengde Medical College*, 2007(2): 189–191.

[265] Qin Li, Hong Liu, Bingzhi Li, *et al.* Pharmacological action and clinical application of Shenmai Injection. *Medical Recapitulate*, 2005(12): 1142–1143.

[266] Yanping Duan, Chenglong Meng, Ping Li. Pharmacological action and clinical application of Shenmai Injection. *China Medical Abstracts* (*Medicine*), 2002(5): 698–699.

Index

9 789811 227875

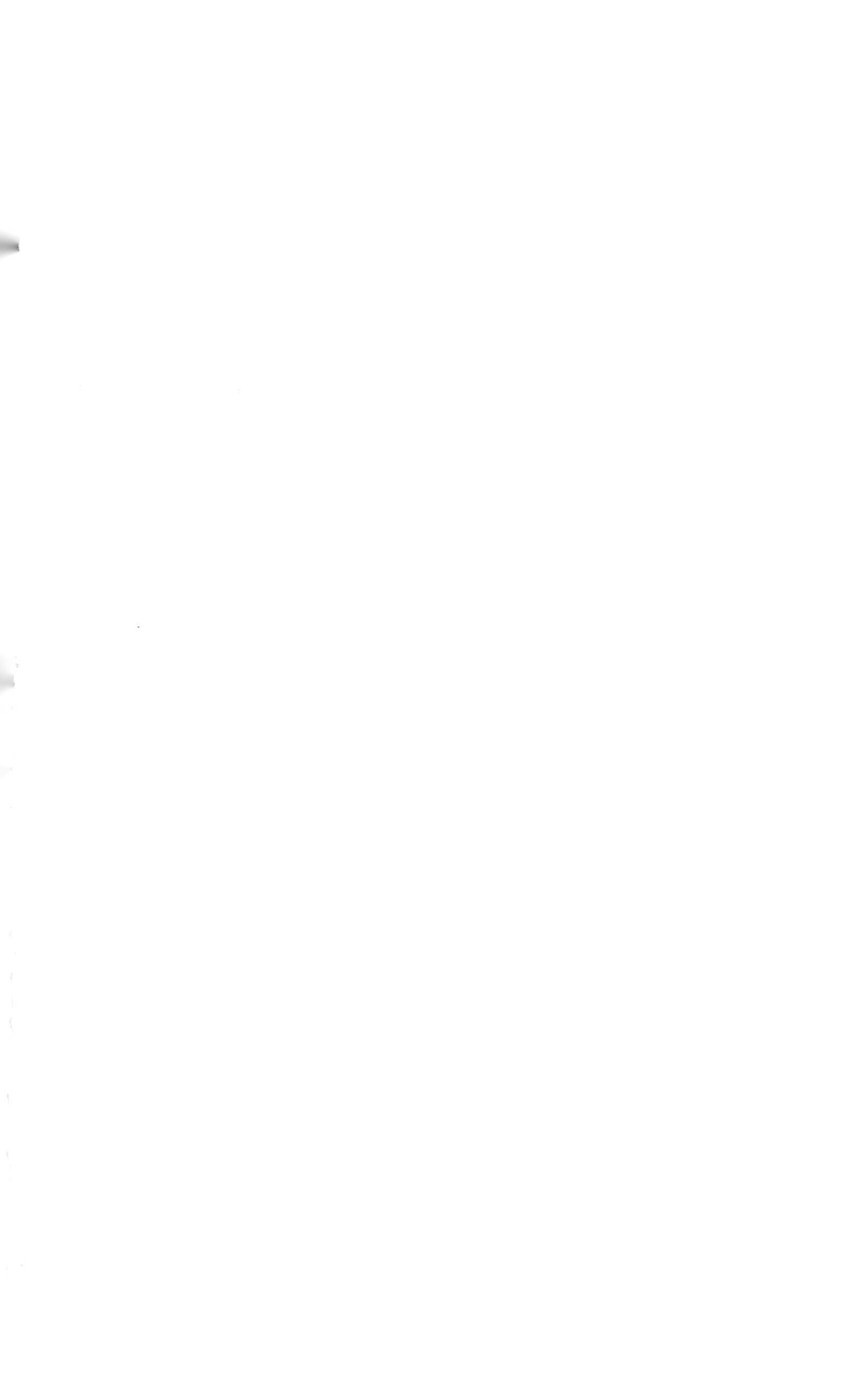